Defeat High Blood Sugar – Naturally!

Super-Supplements and Super-Foods
Selected by America's Best Alternative Doctors

by Bill Gottlieb, CHC

Defeat High Blood Sugar – Naturally!
Super-Supplements and Super-Foods
Selected by America's Best Alternative Doctors

By Bill Gottlieb, CHC

Published by Online Publishing & Marketing, LLC

IMPORTANT CAUTION:

This Special Report is not intended to take the place of medical advice from a trained medical professional. Readers are advised to consult a physician or other qualified health professional regarding treatment of their medical problems. The author and publishers believe the information contained in this book is accurate, but its accuracy cannot be guaranteed. The publishers and author are not responsible for any adverse effects or results from the use of any of the suggestions, preparations or procedures described in this report. As with any medical treatment, results of the treatments described in this report will vary from one person to another. The reader accepts full responsibility for any action he or she takes based on the information contained in this report.

ISBN 978-1-4675-8755-6

Printed in the United States of America.

ABOUT THE AUTHOR

Bill Gottlieb, CHC, is a health coach certified by the American Association of Drugless Practitioners, the author of 12 health books that have sold more than 2 million copies in the U.S. and around the world, and a health journalist whose articles have appeared in many publications, including *Prevention, Men's Health, Health* and *Bottom Line/Health.* From 1976 to 1995 he worked at Rodale, Inc. where, as the editor-in-chief of Rodale Books and Prevention Magazine Books, he conceived and edited health books that sold more than 40 million copies, including *The Doctors Book of Home Remedies* and *New Choices in Natural Healing.*

Bill's 12 authored books include: the self-help health encyclopedia *Alternative Cures* (Rodale), an international, million-copy bestseller that has been translated into five languages; *Maximum Manhood* (Online Publishing & Marketing), about sexual health for middle-aged and older men; *Real Cause, Real Cure* (Rodale), co-authored with Jacob Teitelbaum, MD, a guide to the underlying causes and natural cures for 60 health problems; *Breakthroughs in Natural Healing 2012* and *Breakthroughs in Natural Healing 2011* (both from Bottom Line Publications), featuring reports about new research into drug-free healing; *Speed Healing* (Bottom Line Publications), about fast and natural ways to deal with dozens of diseases and conditions; *Breakthroughs in Drug-Free Healing* (Bottom Line Publications), which reports hundreds of scientific studies on natural remedies; *The Natural Fat-Loss Pharmacy* (Broadway), co-authored with Harry Preuss, MD, about nutritional and herbal supplements to aid fat and weight loss; *The Every-Other-Day Diet,* a revolutionary, science-proven weight loss program that allows you to eat anything you want and all you want, every other day (Hyperion); and *Healing Spices* (Sterling), which Bill conceived, edited and produced through his book packaging company, Good For You Books.

Bill's website is www.billgottliebhealth.com. For inquiries about his health coaching or editorial consulting services, you can email him at bill@billgottliebhealth.com.

Contents

PART I

Diabetes, The Curable Disease

Conventional medicine says diabetes is a life sentence.
Conventional medicine is wrong.

Chapter 1

We Beat Diabetes—Without Drugs!

Inspiring stories from the front lines of natural healing

Talk to 9 out of 10 doctors about diabetes—no, make that 99 out of 100—and they'll tell you that a diabetes diagnosis is set in stone: once you have the disease, you'll *always* have the disease. And it's bound to get worse.

Don't listen to them.

"I have worked with thousands of diabetic patients," I was told by Julian Whitaker, MD, author of *Reversing Diabetes* and medical director of the Whitaker Wellness Institute in Newport Beach, California. "Rather than relying on lifelong drug regimens, we instruct our patients about dietary measures, exercise and nutritional supplements that lower blood sugar as effectively as drugs. We teach them to effectively *reverse* diabetes.

"Most of us are taught that diabetes is not *reversible*—and that we are destined to suffer progressive decline in function, including heart disease, kidney failure, blindness, amputations, strokes and dementia," said Mark Hyman, MD, author of *The Blood Sugar Solution* and chairman of the Institute for Functional Medicine.

"However," he told me, "it is clear from the scientific literature that diabetes *is* reversible—especially if it is caught in the early stages and treated aggressively through lifestyle intervention and nutritional support, and occasionally with medications. Even most later-stage diabetes can be reversed with very intensive lifestyle changes, supplements and medications."

Many of the *former* diabetes patients I talked with while writing *Defeat High Blood Sugar – Naturally* are living proof of what these two doctors (and many more) are saying. I think you'll be inspired by some of their stories.

(In the next chapter—"What Is Diabetes?"—I define many of the diabetes-related terms you'll read here, and also talk about the causes and complications of this 21st century epidemic. But these first-person stories are so inspiring about the effectiveness of drugless treatments for blood sugar problems —and so *shocking* about the ineffectiveness and dangers of the conventional approach—that I wanted you to read them first thing.)

"I can't believe these numbers are so low. What did you do?"

"I was diagnosed with type 2 diabetes on September 23, 2011," said the efficient, to-the-point email from Andy Pattantyus, a 55-year-old mechanical engineer in Santa Clarita, California. Andy wrote me after I put a notice on an internet site asking to hear from folks who'd reversed their diabetes with all-natural, drugless treatments.

"I rejected all the advice offered by the American Diabetes Association and Kaiser Permanente," he continued. "Instead, I did my own research and designed my own drugless program. Following my own regimen, my A1C [a measurement of long-term blood sugar levels] went from 10.3 in September, 2011…to 5.7 in December, 2011…and to 4.7 by April, 2012." (5.7 to 6.4 is prediabetes; 6.5 and above is diabetes.)

Intrigued, I called Andy and asked him to tell me about his diagnosis of diabetes—and how he reversed the disease with drug-free methods.

"I had made a doctor's appointment because I was feeling crappy," he told me. "After looking at my blood work, the doctor said, 'You're a diabetic.' I said, 'Are you sure?' And she said, 'Positively, absolutely, unequivocally certain.'

"Then she started typing a prescription into a computer, and I asked, 'What are you doing?' And she said, 'Writing prescriptions for pills.' And I said, 'What pills?' And she said, 'Metformin—we start all diabetics out on that pill. And terazosin, to help out with frequent urination. And Coumadin, for blood-thinning.' And I'm sent down to the pharmacy and come home with a bag full of drugs.

"Well, I put all that stuff on the kitchen table, and I said to myself, 'It's crap—crap, crap, crap.' And I thought, 'I don't know if this thing is *reversible*—but if it is, that's my goal. And my other goal was to handle it with nutrition and exercise, and ditch the pills as soon as possible.

"You see, I'm a mechanical engineer—a systems thinker. To an engineer like me, every problem is a solvable problem. You create a big picture, plan what you want to accomplish, and deal with the details one by one, until you execute the plan." And that's just what Andy did with his diabetes.

He researched, plowing through "40 of the best books on diabetes and nutrition," and decided what to eat. He started walking, because he'd always enjoyed it. He put some herbs and super-foods in his diet, like a teaspoon of cinnamon on his morning (whole-grain, steel-cut) oatmeal, along with hemp seeds, flax meal and a banana. He found out he was vitamin D deficient, started taking a high-dose vitamin D pill once a week, and now takes 5,000 IU daily. (In Chapter 12, you'll discover why the nationwide epidemic of vitamin D deficiency and the epidemic of diabetes are closely linked—and exactly how much vitamin D you need to help prevent or reverse diabetes.)

And he shocked his doctors.

"I have a different doctor with each visit, and each one expresses amazement over what has happened," he told me. "They say, 'I can't believe these numbers are so low—what did you do?' And for the 10 to 15 minutes of my appointment, I tell them what I did—and they furiously type notes. Better than typing in another prescription, don't you think?"

"Doctors said I would need insulin for the rest of my life —but they didn't know what they were talking about."

Elizabeth Mwanga, a 36-year-old in Queens Village, New York, is the founder of the company WINNING DIABETICS™. Here is her inspiring story of drugless healing…

"In 2007, at the age of 31, I was diagnosed with diabetes," she told me. "I'm 5'1", and in 2004 I weighed 150 pounds. But I had a stressful breakup…ate too much, including a lot of fast food, which I love…and in 2007 weighed 205 and had all the symptoms of diabetes—thirst, urinating a lot, fatigue, constant hunger, vision problems…

"I ended up in the emergency room with diabetic ketoacidosis, a severe and acute form of diabetes. My glucose levels were 1,000, nearly ten times normal. I was in intensive care for four days, on an insulin drip.

"When I was discharged, I was prescribed injectable insulin, to be taken four times daily— and my doctors told me I would remain on insulin for the rest of my life. But they didn't know what they were talking about.

"After 19 months of *drugless* treatment—mostly cutting out carbohydrates and adding exercise—I was able to lose 100 pounds—and have been medicine-free since 2009. At the age of 36, I am in the best shape and health of my life.

"I truly know and believe in my heart that you can regulate blood sugar without drugs. And if *I* can figure out that drugless treatment works—and I've never been to medical school— why can't *doctors* figure it out? But they will, because it's the best way. I'm sure that *lifestyle* management of diabetes is the next generation of treatment."

Taking six drugs for diabetes—and none of them worked

"I can't offer you a medical opinion about diabetes, because I'm not a doctor," wrote Jay Estis, a business consultant in southern Florida. "But I can offer you the perspective of a 51-year-old man whose diabetes was out-of-control—and who has normal blood sugar today, thanks to diet and exercise."

"I was diagnosed with diabetes four years ago, and my doctor at the time immediately prescribed Avandia," Jay told me when we talked on the phone. "Still in shock from learning I had a chronic disease, I went home and Googled the name of the drug and was horrified by what I found." (He's referring to a study which showed that people who took Avandia had a 27% higher risk of stroke, a 25% higher risk of heart failure and a 14% higher risk of death than those taking a similar diabetes drug.)

"I immediately found a new doctor, who prescribed metformin," he continued. "During the first 18 months of my treatment, everything seemed fine—I adjusted my diet to include fewer carbs, took metformin, and felt okay. But then, without any warning or obvious cause, my blood sugar began to spike. And the doctor prescribed a second oral medication.

"Well, it didn't control the situation. My blood sugar spiked even higher, and I was feeling awful all the time—I woke up feeling like I hadn't slept for four days, and I struggled to work for just 5 or 10 minutes without feeling like I needed to lie down and go to sleep. At that point, my doctor prescribed a *third* oral medication.

"I continued to feel bad for nearly a year. Finally, on a holiday weekend, I started to feel even worse, which I didn't think was possible. I knew my blood sugar was rising again and, because my doctor wasn't available, I went to a walk-in clinic. My blood sugar was over 400! They gave me a shot of insulin, and monitored me until my blood sugar normalized.

"During my follow-up visit to my primary care doctor, I was prescribed injectable insulin, which I started injecting three times a day into my stomach, along with taking the oral medications. After a couple of months, I saw an endocrinologist at the University of Miami, and was given another type of insulin—and I also continued with my oral medication regimen, at higher and higher doses. But I wasn't feeling any better—and I was gaining a lot of weight.

"I was never told by a single medical doctor that my diabetes was reversible."

"So one day I sat down at my computer and began doing my *own* research. My first, shocking discovery was that insulin was the cause of the 30 pounds of weight gain I had experienced since starting the drug. I also learned that weight gain from insulin is a vicious cycle that causes you to need *more* of the drug…and you gain more weight…and need more insulin… and so on.

"But perhaps the most shocking and disturbing thing I learned during this time of self-education was that I had never been told by a single medical doctor that my diabetes was totally *reversible*. Nor did a single doctor discuss with me using anti-diabetes supplements or super-foods.

"Over the course of the next several months I found another doctor, and demanded he wean me off insulin.

"I also started taking supplements recommended for diabetes by leading nutritional doctors, including a multivitamin and mineral supplement, vitamin D, omega-3 fish oil, alpha-lipoic acid, chromium, biotin, cinnamon, and PGX, a fiber supplement."

(You'll find crucial information about all these supplements—what they are; how they work; and how to put them to work for you—throughout this Special Report. Vitamin D is featured in Chapter 12…omega-3 fish oil in Chapter 13…alpha-lipoic acid in Chapter 14…chromium and biotin in Chapter 11…cinnamon in Chapter 16…and PGX in Chapter 5.)

"And," said Jay, "I started educating myself about the power of whole foods and super-foods like cacao powder [dark chocolate], goji berry powder and flaxseeds, gradually introducing them into my diet. Now, I include them in my diet every day."

(Ditto for the lowdown on dark chocolate: you can read about its amazing heart-protective powers in Chapter 25.)

"Since starting my super-foods diet, I have lost the 30 pounds I gained on insulin, plus an additional 15…am completely off injectable insulin…and I have stopped taking all my oral drugs, except for metformin. I expect to stop taking that, too, when I have completely reversed my diabetes.

"Also, I recently added daily exercise to my routine, which I am sure will speed up the reversal process. In brief, I went from months of being barely able to function—to feeling better than I have in years!

"Doctors only tell you that you can 'manage' diabetes, and that the only way to do it is with medication. But diabetes can be *reversed*.

"It is so important to get this story of natural diabetes cures out there, so people understand what their options are—and that what your doctor tells you to do for diabetes might *not* be the best for you."

Myth: diabetes is a genetic disease

Jay told me that he thought his diabetes could have been prevented—if only he'd been given better advice sooner.

"My mother was diabetic prior to her passing. My father was an insulin-diabetic ever since I was a kid. My sister was diagnosed with type 2 diabetes. So, of course, doctors heard my family history, and looked at my blood work, and told me it was only a matter of time until I became diabetic, too—and they would start to treat me when my time came. The problem with that kind of thinking? It's completely *false*. I developed my diabetes because of my *lifestyle*—not because of genes—and I reversed it because of my *lifestyle*."

Supplements reversed her heart disease

Janice O. is a 62-year-old paralegal in northern California. Her 82-year-old mother, who lives nearby, is an insulin-dependent diabetes patient, and Janice has seen firsthand just how difficult life has become for her mom as her diabetes has advanced over the last 20 years. That's why Janice "freaked out" when her yearly physical in 2008 showed her A1C was in the prediabetes range.

"I read all the books I could on diabetes, and began eating a low-glycemic index diet, exercising regularly and taking nutritional supplements," she told me. "I really didn't want my A1C to get any worse!"

But while her A1C levels stayed fairly low, her most recent physical showed that her risk factors for heart disease were definitely getting riskier—her LDL cholesterol was 151 (borderline high)…her total cholesterol was 265 (high)…and her triglycerides were 217 (high).

Fortunately for Janice, she was under the care of a natural-minded doctor—who changed her supplement regimen to lower those numbers, adding or increasing the dosage of many of the supplements you'll be reading about in this Special Report, including Coenzyme Q10, vitamin D, and omega-3 fatty acids. He also put her on red yeast rice, an herbal statin. "I took these supplements religiously," she told me. And a miracle occurred.

After just three months, her LDL fell to 98 (optimal)…her total cholesterol was at 197 (desirable)…and her triglycerides plummeted to 70 (normal).

"I am so happy that I controlled my heart disease risk factors *naturally* with supplements and other non-drug treatments, and did not have to go on Lipitor or any other medications," Janice told me.

In the next chapter...

These amazing stories (and many more like them that you'll read throughout this Special Report) are proof-positive that diabetes is not merely "controllable" but *reversible*—using super-supplements, super-foods and other natural therapies. In the next chapter, we'll take a closer look at the disease itself: how many of us have prediabetes or diabetes…why the incidence of the disease is skyrocketing…and its terrible complications. (Then it's just about time to start preventing or reversing the problem!)

EXPERTS AND CONTRIBUTORS:

Jay Estis is a business consultant in southern Florida who reversed his diabetes using a natural program of self-care.

Mark Hyman, MD, was co-medical director of Canyon Ranch for almost 10 years and is now the chairman of the Institute for Functional Medicine and founder and medical director of the UltraWellness Center. He is the *New York Times* bestselling author of *UltraMetabolism, The UltraMind Solution*, and the *UltraSimple Diet*.
Websites: www.drhyman.com, www.bloodsugarsolution.com
Facebook: facebook.com/drmarkhyman
Twitter: @markhymanmd

Elizabeth Mwanga is the founder of WINNING DIABETICS™. She is a Healthy Food blogger for AOL Black Voices. She has been featured in *Redbook, Woman's Day, Ebony, NY Newsday* and *More*, and her diabetic-friendly recipes have been featured on The Dr. Oz Show.
Website: www.winningdiabetics.com
Facebook: www.facebook.com/winningdiabetics
Twitter: @winningdiabetics

Janice O. is a paralegal in northern California.

Andy Pattantyus, the President of Strategic Modularity, Inc. in Santa Clarita, California, reversed his diabetes using natural therapies.
Website: www.strategicmodularity.com

Julian Whitaker, MD, is author of *Reversing Diabetes: Reduce Or Even Eliminate Your Dependence On Insulin Or Oral Drugs*, and medical director of the Whitaker Wellness Institute in Newport Beach, California.
Website: www.drwhitaker.com

Chapter 2

What Is Diabetes?

Prediabetes and diabetes are destroying the health of 105 million Americans. If you understand the disease, you can protect yourself.

If you're an adult American, it's pretty likely you have diabetes or prediabetes. That's because…

105 million Americans have problems with high blood sugar.

An estimated 79 million Americans have *prediabetes*—blood sugar readings of 100 to 125 mg/dl. (Shockingly, a study conducted by researchers at the Centers for Disease Control and Prevention revealed that 93% of people with prediabetes *don't know* they have the condition. That might include you.)

And prediabetes is *serious*.

"Prediabetes is not 'pre' anything," I was told by Mark Hyman, MD, author of *The Blood Sugar Solution*. "It is a deadly disease driving our biggest killers—heart attacks, strokes, cancer, dementia and more. It carries with it nearly all the risks of diabetes."

Another 26 million have *diabetes***,** with nearly all of them suffering from type 2 diabetes—blood sugar readings of 126 mg/dl or higher. (Twenty-seven percent of people with type 2 diabetes don't know they have it.)

And those numbers are going up. Way up. In 1980, 5 million Americans had diabetes. In 1990, the number had risen to 7 million. By 2000, it was 12 million. By 2005, 16 million. Today, it's 26 million. And researchers are predicting that by 2025 more than 50 million Americans will have diabetes.

Seniors are hardest hit. Two out of every three Americans over 65 has either prediabetes or diabetes.

But nowadays even kids are affected: the percentage of teens with prediabetes or diabetes has more than doubled, from 9% in 1999 to 23% today. One out of every four American teenagers has a condition that hardly even existed among teens 30 years ago! It's deeply shocking that this "disease of aging" has now become a childhood disease!

What's behind this raging epidemic?

The many causes of high blood sugar

Many factors are causing the rapid increase of prediabetes and diabetes in America and around the world. They include…

Being overweight. Four out of five people who have prediabetes and diabetes are also overweight. (Some experts call the problem *diabesity*.) That's because fat cells don't just sit there. They generate compounds that create *oxidation* (a kind of cellular rust) and low-grade, chronic, body-wide *inflammation*.

Oxidation and inflammation—the evil twins of chronic disease—make your cells *insulin resistant*: they no longer respond easily and naturally to insulin, the hormone that moves glucose out of the bloodstream and into cells. Extra fat also clogs insulin receptors on cells, increasing insulin resistance.

At first, the beta-cells of your pancreas pump out more insulin (which is also inflammatory). Eventually, your exhausted beta-cells start to die—and you have to take oral insulin or insulin injections just to stay alive.

Body fat—particularly the extra belly fat that surrounds and invades glucose-regulating organs like the pancreas and liver—is the foundation of high blood sugar. But it's not the whole building.

Eating too much sugar and other refined carbs. The average American eats 150 pounds of *added* sugar per year—in sugary beverages, cookies, cakes and even in foods like ketchup, since sugar is added routinely to most processed foods. We also eat a lot of refined carbohydrates from white bread, chips and other high-carb foods.

All those quick-digesting carbohydrates flood your bloodstream with glucose, taxing your poor pancreas until it cries Uncle. Sugar and other refined carbs also cause inflammation and oxidation, increasing insulin resistance.

The newest research: Every additional 150 calories in sugar that you eat per day (the amount in one soda) raises your risk of diabetes by 1%—ten times higher than the risk created by consuming an additional 150 calories of any other food. We're literally killing ourselves with sugar.

Nutritional deficiencies. As you'll read in this Special Report, a diet lacking in certain essential nutrients—like magnesium and vitamin D—is a setup for prediabetes and diabetes. And with so many empty calories from sugar and fat, the American diet is woefully lacking in vitamins and minerals.

Lack of exercise. A no-exercise lifestyle is a setup for blood sugar problems. That's because fit muscles have cells that are *insulin sensitive*—they easily use glucose, clearing it out of the bloodstream. But the cells of unfit muscles are insulin resistant—and blood glucose stays high.

Poor sleep. Lack of sleep can exhaust your body's ability to manage glucose—studies show sleep problems *triple* your risk of developing diabetes. And sleep apnea—when the soft tissue at the back of your throat obstructs your airway, cutting off breathing and rousing you to a semi-awake state many times during the night—doubles your risk of diabetes. (28 million Americans—mostly middle-aged and older men—have sleep apnea.)

Constant stress. Non-stop stress puts your endocrine system into "fight-or-flight" overdrive, generating hormones that boost blood sugar.

The newest research: If you have "permanent stress" at home or work, you are 45% more likely to develop diabetes.

Prescription drugs. This next one is a shocker: Many commonly prescribed drugs increase your risk for prediabetes and diabetes—including cholesterol-lowering statins…beta-blockers used to control high blood pressure, irregular heart beat and heart failure…antidepressants and anti-psychotics…ACE inhibitors for high blood pressure…and the alpha-blockers prescribed for high blood pressure and prostate problems.

Pollutants. Recent studies link pollutants—from heavy metals like lead and cadmium, to "persistent organic pollutants" like pesticides—to an increased risk for diabetes. The pollutants might directly damage the pancreas. Or they might damage the intestinal tract, leading to chronic inflammation.

The newest research: If you have high blood levels of a persistent organic pollution like a pesticide, you are four times more likely to develop diabetes!

Genes. If you have a family history of diabetes, all of the risk factors you just read about are even riskier for you.

As you can see (and as so many of us have unfortunately discovered) *modern life*—the diet, the sitting, the stress and lack of sleep, the medications, the pollution—is the cause of the epidemic of prediabetes and type 2 diabetes. And this epidemic of blood sugar problems means there's also an epidemic of suffering…

High blood sugar destroys your health

High blood sugar slowly but surely destroys your circulatory system—from the rivers of your arteries to the cell-by-cell trickle of the capillaries.

Also, people with prediabetes and the early stages of type 2 diabetes usually have high blood levels of *insulin*, the hormone that guides glucose out of the bloodstream and into cells. High insulin levels are toxic, too. Consider these frightening facts about the destructive power of diabetes…

Heart attacks and strokes. If you have diabetes, you have up to *four times* the risk of having a heart attack or stroke—the cause of death of 84% of people with diabetes.

Alzheimer's disease. Likewise, if you have diabetes, you have *four times* the risk of Alzheimer's disease, as a flood of glucose and insulin batters the cells of the brain.

Nerve damage. About two-thirds of people with diabetes develop *peripheral neuropathy*—nerve damage in the feet and hands, with pain, burning, shock-like tingling, itching and numbness.

Amputations. Poor circulation to the feet often leads to skin ulcers that don't heal and become infected. Eventually, amputation is the only option: diabetes is the leading cause of amputations in the U.S. that aren't the result of an accident—67,000 amputations a year.

Failing eyesight. The tiny blood vessels that feed the retina at the back of the eye become diseased, leading to *diabetic retinopathy*—and to poor vision and eventual blindness. Thirty percent of people with diabetes have vision problems, and diabetes is the #1 cause of new cases of blindness in American adults. (Diabetes also damages the proteins in the lens of the eye, increasing your risk of cataracts.)

Kidney failure. Too much blood glucose damages the tiny blood vessels of the kidney, leading to *diabetic nephropathy*, which further stresses your circulatory system. (New research shows that diabetic nephropathy dramatically increases the risk of heart attack and stroke in diabetes patients.) Diabetes is the most common cause of the more than 200,000 yearly cases of chronic kidney failure in the U.S.—an organ failure that requires either dialysis (getting your blood cleaned by a machine three times a week) or a kidney transplant.

Premature aging—and early death. And diabetes just flat out *ages* you. All that extra glucose binds with proteins to form toxic molecules called, appropriately enough, AGEs—advanced glycation end products. AGEs ruin the youthful tone of every organ and part of your body, from your skin to your bone marrow, and they're a main reason why diabetes is so deadly. How deadly, exactly? A 50-year-old with diabetes has an average lifespan 8.5 years shorter than a

50-year-old without the illness. And in any given year, a person with diabetes is *twice* as likely to die as someone who doesn't have the disease.

Talking about diabetes: defining some technical terms

As doctors test and treat high blood sugar and its complications, they use a lot of technical terms—and since I'll be using some of them throughout this Special Report, I'd like to define them right off. For example, blood glucose levels are tested in several ways.

There's the ***fasting plasma glucose test***—a measurement taken first thing in the morning before eating, or eight hours after your most recent meal. Two fasting glucose tests of 126 mg/dl or higher result in a diagnosis of type 2 diabetes. If you test from 100 to 125, you've got prediabetes.

Another test is **A1C**—***glycated hemoglobin***. (It's also called *glycosolated hemoglobin*, in case you hear that term.) This test measures the percentage of red blood cells frosted with glucose. And since red blood cells live for three months, the test reveals your average blood sugar levels during that time period.

An A1C of 5.6% or lower is normal…5.7 to 6.4% is prediabetes…and 6.5% or higher is type 2 diabetes.

Another test for diabetes is the ***oral glucose tolerance test***. You drink a big dose of glucose and the doctor measures blood sugar levels every 30 minutes or so for the next three hours. In that test, 140 to 200 mg/dl is prediabetes, and over 200 is diabetes. If you have prediabetes based on this test, a doctor might say you have *poor glucose tolerance* or are *glucose intolerant*.

Doctors sometimes measure ***postprandial glucose***, taking your blood sugar levels one to two hours after a meal. Big post-meal spikes in glucose (higher than 140, according to the American College of Endocrinology) are a sure sign of poor blood sugar control. And those spikes, because they trigger an avalanche of oxidation and inflammation, are also a risk factor for heart disease.

You might also come across the term ***metabolic syndrome***, which has five different definitions, depending on the health organization doing the defining. (The American Heart Association, the International Diabetes Federation, The World Health Organization, etc.)

Basically, metabolic syndrome is a bunch of health problems that hang out together like a gang, threatening your health: high blood sugar (in the prediabetes range); extra belly fat; high blood pressure; low HDL cholesterol; and high triglycerides. Metabolic syndrome increases your risk for heart disease and diabetes. But many health professionals I interviewed for this Special

Report think it's not all that useful as a diagnosis. So I mostly use the terms "prediabetes" and "diabetes," except when I'm reporting on a scientific study that focuses on metabolic syndrome.

This report does not address two other kinds of diabetes: *type 1 diabetes* (an autoimmune disease that attacks the pancreas, and afflicts 1.3 million Americans); and *gestational diabetes* (occurring in about one out of six pregnancies; many women with the problem develop type 2 diabetes within 10 years).

In this Special Report, I focus on the most common blood sugar problems: **prediabetes and type 2 diabetes**. When I refer to "diabetes" I mean type 2 diabetes.

In the next chapter...

Now you know what diabetes is…what it does to you…and what doctors are talking about when they diagnose and treat the disease. In the next chapter, we'll take a close look at the conventional approach to high blood sugar—drugs, drugs and more drugs—and why those medications are often nothing more than "band aids" that do nothing to heal the problem—and can also trigger a whole set of *new* health problems (including very serious diseases like heart attack, stroke and cancer).

Chapter 3

The Slippery Slope of Diabetes Drugs

Are drugs for diabetes sometimes worse than the disease?
These doctors think so.

You'd think a pharmacist would be the last person to have second thoughts about taking a medication for blood sugar problems. That is, until you talk to Curtis Alexander, PharmD, a pharmacist in Montana who used drugless methods—*not* drugs—to reverse his prediabetes.

"When I was 35, I was gaining weight, feeling sluggish, and had unexplained rashes," he told me. "Since both my grandmothers were diabetic, and one of my parents was recently put on a metformin to control her blood sugar, I decided to get my glucose levels checked, to see if they might have something to do with how bad I felt. I took a glucose tolerance test—and after the test the doctor told me that I was prediabetic!

"Honestly, it took me a few years to take that diagnosis seriously—to research diabetes in depth and find out how to *really* deal with it. And what I discovered is that the best way to reverse the problem was *without* drugs—and that's what I did. Now, my fasting blood sugar is 85 to 90, well within the normal range."

But he's a *pharmacist*. Why didn't he just pop a pill for glucose control? I asked.

"In almost every case, prescription drugs are *not* the real answer to chronic health problems, and that includes diabetes," he answered passionately. "Drugs are *band aids*—and generally poor ones. They treat the *symptoms*, not the cause—they don't get to the *root* of the problem."

"I don't care *what* drug you're taking for diabetes," he continued. "If you're taking a drug for the disease, you're headed down the wrong path. Drugless healing—nutritional healing—is the way to *really* deal with diabetes."

A lot of other health professionals share his perspective about drugs and diabetes.

"Avoid drugs whenever possible."

"People with blood sugar problems should *avoid* drugs whenever possible," said Julian Whitaker, MD, medical director of the Whitaker Wellness Institute in Newport Beach, California.

"The intensive use of oral diabetes drugs has been linked to serious health problems," he told me. "And harmful side effects have also been linked to drugs used to treat high blood pressure and heart disease, which are common in diabetes patients. The more you minimize the need for medication—by using natural approaches to blood sugar control and circulatory health—the better."

Are you on the medication merry-go-round?

"If the readers of your Special Report have prediabetes or diabetes, and currently don't take medications, they should do all they can to avoid taking them," I was told by Suzy Cohen, RPh, a licensed pharmacist, and author of *Diabetes Without Drugs*.

"Once your physician orders medication for diabetes, you start on what I call the 'medication merry-go-round,'" she said. "You take one medication, and it sparks side effects— because it steals your nutrients, a condition I call 'drug mugging,' in which a new drug robs the body of vital nutrients.

"The supposed 'side effects'—really caused by nutrient depletion—will then be diagnosed as *new* diseases, and you will receive *more* drugs to deal with these new 'symptoms.'

"Years may pass as you sit on this merry-go-round—going around in circles, never moving forward—while the underlying problem is never fixed!

"Sure, drugs can bring your blood sugar numbers down. But if you're taking medications without using drugless natural approaches—like diet, supplements and exercise—your pancreas continues to die, one cell at a time, and inflammatory chemicals cause more damage and pain.

"Popular diabetes medications don't address these *causes* of ongoing blood sugar problems. Most diabetes drugs—aside from insulin, which is useful if you have type 1 diabetes or severe type 2 diabetes—only cover up symptoms. They don't reduce inflammation or reverse the disease."

Limited benefits, significant risks

"Drugless approaches—nutrition, supplements, exercise and stress reduction—always work much more quickly and dramatically than medications for diabetes," I was told by Mark Hyman, MD, chairman of the Institute for Functional Medicine.

(Dr. Hyman, Dr. Whitaker and the other remarkable, natural-minded clinicians I've featured in these first few chapters are colleagues and friends, with excellent programs and products for blood sugar control. But I have to say that in researching this Special Report I found some super-supplements and super-foods even they don't know about. In fact, these natural solutions are *so* powerful, you can literally manage diabetes without drugs *and* without the lifestyle changes like diet and exercise that we both know you should make. Now back to the downside of drugs for diabetes…)

"The only diabetes medication that I find helpful is metformin, or Glucophage," Dr. Hyman writes. "It is well tolerated, has been around a long time, and has been well studied. Most of the other medications cause serious complications or make things worse by boosting insulin levels and increasing the risk of death and heart attacks. Yes, other doctors prescribe these medications—but they have limited benefits and significant risks. That is why I stay away from most of them."

Let's put the spotlight on some of those "serious complications" and "significant risks" so you can see for yourself exactly what Dr. Hyman is talking about…

Byetta and Januvia: Is their "side effect" cancer?

Millions of Americans with diabetes now take one of the newest diabetes drugs: Januvia (sitagliptin) or Byetta (exenatide).

These drugs either increase or preserve levels of the gut hormone GLP-1 (glucagon-like peptide-1), which triggers the pancreas to pump out more insulin. In many cases, the pancreas isn't too happy about it.

A 2013 study shows that people taking Januvia or Byetta have twice the risk of hospitalization for *pancreatitis*—inflammation of the pancreas, with nausea, non-stop vomiting and abdominal pain. [1] But an inflamed pancreas is a cakewalk compared to another risk from these drugs: pancreatic cancer.

A study by researchers at UCLA found nearly *three times* more pancreatic cancer among people using Januvia or Byetta. [2] (They also found a six-fold increase in pancreatitis, compared to people taking other types of diabetes drugs.)

To add insult to pancreatic injury, Januvia and Byetta might not be doing you any good.

Dr. Hyman points to a large study showing these drugs don't reduce the health risks of diabetes—and that after one year of taking the drug most diabetes patients had *higher* levels of insulin and glucose. "I avoid prescribing these drugs," he said.

NEWS FLASH: In May 2013, as this Special Report was in production, a doctor at UCLA declared in an online version of the journal *Diabetes Care* that Januvia and similar drugs (incretins) definitely predispose people taking them to pancreatic cancer. "The safety" of these drugs, he wrote, "can no longer be assumed." He continued...

"The story is familiar. A new class of antidiabetic agents is rushed to market and widely promoted in the absence of any evidence of long-term beneficial outcomes. Evidence of harm accumulates, but is vigorously discounted. The regulators allow years to pass before they act. The manufacturers are expected--quite unrealistically--to monitor the safety of their own product."

Bottom line: Another popular class of diabetes drugs is declared unsafe--while safe, natural options for blood sugar control abound!

Avandia and Actos: Caution—heart attacks ahead

The story of the diabetes drug Avandia (rosiglitazone)—once the top-selling diabetes drug in the world—is a story of deception, greed and thousands of unnecessary deaths.

48,000, to be exact.

That's the number of deaths from heart disease caused by Avandia, from the time it came on the market in 1999, until 2010, when evidence for its deadly risks became overwhelming, and its use was banned in Europe and limited in the U.S.

But the infuriating fact is that the drug's manufacturer, GlaxoSmithKline (GSK), *knew* in 1999 that Avandia could hurt the heart—and spent the next 11 years covering up the truth! That profit-over-patient perspective was summed up in an email written by a drug company executive: "These data [about Avandia] should not see the light of day to anyone outside GSK."

Well, they did see the light of day. And in 2012 GlaxoSmithKline pleaded guilty to criminal charges that it had failed to report the safety data about Avandia (as well as several other illegalities, like giving doctors kickbacks to prescribe drugs)—and paid a fine of $3 billion dollars.

(Avandia is so bad, even some doctors are fed up with it. The story of Avandia, said an editorial in the *British Medical Journal* "says much about how healthcare has become less about promoting patients' interests, alleviating illness, and curing disease, and more about promoting the interests of the drug industry.")

Needless to say, Avandia isn't prescribed much these days: only 3,400 patients take the severely restricted drug

But that's not true of Actos (pioglitazone), its sibling in the family of drugs called *thiazolidinediones*, which work by decreasing insulin resistance. There are 15 million yearly prescriptions for Actos in the U.S. And that's unfortunate, because *neither* drug is safe.

Both drugs nearly triple the risk of eye problems and vision loss in diabetes, reported a study in the *American Journal of Ophthalmology*. [3]

Both drugs increase the risk of bone fractures in people 50 and older, according to five studies published from 2008 to 2010—with one study showing they double the risk of fractures in women. [4]

Both drugs double or triple the risk of bladder cancer, according to research funded by the National Institutes of Health. [5]

NEWS FLASH: Just when you thought it was be safe to go back in the pharmacy again, Avandia has reared its ugly side effects. As this Special Report was in production, 20 of 26 panelists on an FDA advisory committee recommended easing the restrictions on Avandia. And that's after 10 members of another panel voted to *ban* the drug in 2010! (Makes you wonder how many of those pro-Avandia panel members are also paid consultants for drug companies.)

And here's another late-breaking shocker: just one month after the FDA advisory panel kowtowed to Avandia, the drug company Roche stopped the development of aleglitazer, a medication in the same class of diabetes drugs as Avandia. Why? Because in a clinical trial the drug increased fractures, kidney problems and heart failure.

This clinical trial "shows that the class of drugs has significant problems with toxicity, particularly cardiovascular toxicity," Steven E. Nissen, MD, the chair of cardiovascular medicine at the Cleveland Clinic (and a big critic of Avandia), told the *New York Times*.

I'd say Dr. Nissen has summed up the situation quite well: Avandia and drugs like it are *toxic*.

In almost all cases, natural remedies are harmless, healthful and truly healing.

Sulfonylureas: One is less deadly than the others

This category of drugs (including glipizide, glyburide, glimepiride) has been around for decades, and works by stimulating the pancreas to produce more insulin. But a recent study links all three sulfonylureas to a 50% greater risk of death, compared to metformin. [6] And if you already have heart disease, glipizide boosts your risk of death by 41% and glyburide by 38%.

(Glimepiride didn't increase the risk of death from heart disease, which makes it slightly superior to the other two, but only because it's slightly less deadly.)

Insulin: The last resort

A 2013 study—conducted over 12 years, and involving more than 84,000 people—showed that diabetes patients on insulin had a...

- 96% increased risk of heart attack

- 43% increased risk of stroke

- 43% increased risk of cancer

- 2.2 times the risk of dying from any cause

- 3.5 times the risk of kidney problems

- 2.1 times the risk of neuropathy

- 17% increased risk of eye problems

"...there are increased health risks for patients with type 2 diabetes who take insulin to manage their condition," concluded the researchers. [7]

"Insulin is the last resort, after all other measures have failed," said Dr. Hyman.

The drugless alternative

Compare the deadly side effects of diabetes drugs to the super-supplements you're going to discover in this Special Report.

There is no comparison. Prescription drugs kill an estimated 100,000 Americans yearly (according to one study in the *New England Journal of Medicine*), with many doctors telling me the real number is probably two or even three times higher.

Well, in 2010 (the most recent year with official data available) there were *zero* deaths from nutritional supplements.

That's right: zero, none, nada.

"If vitamin and mineral supplements are allegedly so 'dangerous' as the FDA and news media so often claim, then where are the bodies?" asked an article in *Orthomolecular News Service*, commenting on the numbers.

Why are supplements so safe?

"Most drugs work by poisoning enzyme systems, the proteins that spark biochemical processes throughout the body," I was told by Jacob Teitelbaum, MD, a natural-minded physician and my co-author in writing the book *Real Cause, Real Cure*. "In contrast to prescription medications, natural remedies such as nutrients and herbs work *with* bodily systems to help the body heal. In fact, most vitamins and minerals work by *activating* rather than *blocking* enzymes."

But if nutrients and herbs are so wonderful, why aren't they promoted as aggressively as drugs? I asked Dr. Teitelbaum. "It's hard to patent natural products because they're *natural*," he explained. "You can't patent air, water, vitamin D or cinnamon, because they've been around a long time. And if you can't patent it, you can't create an exclusive product that makes billions of dollars for your company. Unfortunately, it's profit—not effectiveness or safety—that drives the culture of 21st century American medicine."

Yes, these drugless remedies are POWERFUL —so talk to your doctor before taking them

The real "risk" for the super-supplements and super-foods in this Special Report is that they actually *work* to lower blood sugar levels—which means you and your physician need to pay close attention to any diabetes medications you're taking, and lower the dose (or eliminate them entirely) if necessary.

Of course, one can never be too safe. For that reason, it's best to take the super-supplements in this Special Report with the approval and guidance of a qualified health professional, hopefully one who is savvy about their use and effectiveness.

And whatever super-supplements you decide to take, it's important to remember that two lifestyle changes will MULTIPLY the power of the supplements when it comes to reversing blood sugar problems:

1. A healthful, *enjoyable* diet (like the one I recommend in Chapter 26); and

2. Regular exercise. (The simplest, best and most effective recommendation: a brisk, 30-minute walk, three to four days a week).

But this Special Report is done with drugs—and I hope you are too, or soon will be! It's time to talk about the amazing super-supplements that can *naturally* prevent, control and reverse your blood sugar problems. In the next chapter—Chapter 4—you'll discover…

• How to cut back on your carbohydrate intake by 66%—*without* eating fewer carbs! (Yes, it's really possible—with a remarkable carb-blocking super-supplement.)

• Participants in this study had a blood sugar drop of 22 points—just by taking a carb-blocker.

• The diabetes-causing foods you could be literally *addicted* to like heroin—without even knowing it!

EXPERTS AND CONTRIBUTORS:

Curtis Anderson, PharmD, is a pharmacist in Montana.
Website: www.ask-curtis.com

Suzy Cohen, RPh, is a licensed pharmacist, author of the "Dear Pharmacist" syndicated column, which reaches 20 million readers nationwide, and author of *Diabetes Without Drugs: The 5-Step Program To Control Blood Sugar Naturally And Prevent Diabetes Complications* and several other books.
Website: www.suzycohen.com
Facebook: www.facebook.com/SuzyCohenRPh
Twitter: www.Twitter.com/suzycohen

Mark Hyman, MD, was co-medical director of Canyon Ranch for almost 10 years and is now the chairman of the Institute for Functional Medicine and founder and medical director of the UltraWellness Center. He is the *New York Times* bestselling author of *UltraMetabolism, The UltraMind Solution*, and the *UltraSimple Diet*.
Websites: www.drhyman.com, www.bloodsugarsolution.com
Facebook: facebook.com/drmarkhyman
Twitter: @markhymanmd

Jacob Teitelbaum, MD, is a board certified internist and Medical Director of the national Fibromyalgia and Fatigue Centers and Chronicity. He is author of the popular free iPhone application *Cures A-Z,* and author of the bestselling book *From Fatigued to Fantastic!*, as well as *Pain Free 1-2-3* (McGraw-Hill), *Three Steps to Happiness: Healing Through Joy* and *Beat Sugar Addiction NOW!*. His newest book is *Real Cause, Real Cure*.
Website: www.endfatigue.com

Julian Whitaker, MD, is author of *Reversing Diabetes: Reduce Or Even Eliminate Your Dependence On Insulin Or Oral Drugs*, and medical director of the Whitaker Wellness Institute in Newport Beach, California.
Website: www.drwhitaker.com

REFERENCES:

1. Singh S, et al. Glucagonlike Peptide 1-Based Therapies and Risk of Hospitalization for Acute Pancreatitis in Type 2 Diabetes Mellitus: A Population-Based Matched Case-Control Study. *JAMA Internal Medicine*, 2013 Feb 25:1-6.

2. Elashoff M, et al. Pancreatitis, Pancreatic, and Thyroid Cancer with Glucagon-Like Peptide-1-Based Therapies. *Gastroenterology*, 2011 Jul;141(1):150-6

3. Fong, DS. Glitazone use associated with diabetic macular edema. *American Journal of Ophthalmology*, 2009 Apr;147(4):583-586.

4. Loke YK, et al. Long-term use of thiazolidinediones and fractures in type 2 diabetes: systematic review and meta-analysis. 2009 Jan 6;180(1):32-9.

5. Mamtani R, et al. Association Between Longer Therapy With Thiazolidinediones and Risk of Bladder Cancer: A Cohort Study. *Journal of the National Cancer Institute*, 2012 Sep 19;104(18):1411-21.

6. Pantalone KM, et al. The Endocrine Society 94th Annual Meeting, 2012.

7. Currie CJ, et al. Important Diabetes-Related Outcomes With Insulin vs. Other Antihyperglycemic Therapies in Type 2 Diabetes. *Journal of Clinical Endocrinology & Metabolism*, 2013 Feb;98(2):668-77.

PART II

21st Century Diabetes Cures

These amazing natural supplements are often more powerful than diabetes drugs.

Chapter 4

Carb-Blockers

Stop carbs before they start.

Remember the days when *fat* was the "heavy" in your daily diet—the macronutrient that health experts said was clogging your arteries and crushing your health?

A *low-fat diet* was the cure for what ailed us, said those same experts. And so a lot of us dutifully cut back on fat. We trimmed steaks, banished butter, guzzled skim milk—and ate carbohydrate-rich foods like there was no tomorrow.

Sadly, for many Americans there *was* no tomorrow.

Because over the last three or four decades—when *low-fat...low-fat...low-fat* was the mealtime mantra taught to us by just about every dietician, nutritionist and doctor—a lot of us got a lot fatter. And sicker. And deader.

Yes, as a nation we *gained* weight on the low-fat diet. Since the 1970s, the number of overweight Americans has risen steadily year by year, with more than 70% of us now either overweight (up to 30 pounds above normal) or obese (more than 30 pounds above normal).

And more of us developed diabetes during those same decades: rates have increased by an astonishing 300% since the 1980s.

And diabetes, as we discussed in Chapter 2, is downright deadly, *quadrupling* the risk of heart attack and stroke.

Low-Fat turned out to be a low blow to our collective health.

What happened? *Carbohydrates* happened...

More carbs, more disease

It turns out—much to the surprise of those nutritional experts—that the heavy in the American diet wasn't fat. It was (and is) *carbohydrates*. Specifically, *refined carbohydrates*, like sugar and white flour. (Refined doesn't mean those carbs mind their manners at the dinner table.

It means that food manufacturers start with a whole food and then *refine* it into a food that puts holes in your health—morphing kernels of corn into high-fructose corn syrup, or kernels of whole wheat into white flour.)

Yes, those of us who listened to the "experts" and subtracted fat from our diets merely added something else—refined carbs. A lot of refined carbs.

One-third of the calories we eat are now from the sugar and white flour added to food during processing, I was told by Jacob Teitelbaum, MD, a holistic physician in Hawaii, author of *Beat Sugar Addiction NOW!* and my co-author of the book *Real Cause, Real Cure.*

Our consumption of high-fructose corn syrup—a particularly toxic sweetener that can drive up blood pressure, raising the risk of heart attack and stroke—has nearly *tripled* in the last 15 years, I was told by Richard J. Johnson, MD, a professor in the Department of Medicine at the University of Colorado, and author of *The Sugar Fix: The High-Fructose Fallout That Is Making You Fat and Sick.* The rate of diabetes increased 45% during the same time period.

At the same time, our intake of sugar from beverages—from sodas, fruit drinks, sweetened ice teas, energy drinks and vitamin water drinks—has *doubled.* And that's double trouble.

Frank Hu, MD, PhD, a professor of nutrition and epidemiology at the Harvard School of Public Health, analyzed dietary data from more than 300,000 people. He found that drinking just *one* sugar-sweetened beverage a day—one can of soda, for example—increased the risk of developing prediabetes by 20% and type 2 diabetes by 26%, compared to folks who drink one or fewer sugar-sweetened beverages per month. [1]

In a recent scientific paper in *Current Diabetes Research*, Dr. Hu summed up the situation: the rise in sugar intake and the rise in the rates of type 2 diabetes are a *statistical match.* [2] In other words, increased sugar intake is the likely cause of our diabetes epidemic.

Even the American Heart Association—longtime champions of low-fat eating—now admits that the sugar in our diets is a cause of disease.

In a recent "Scientific Statement," the AHA pointed out that in *just the last decade* Americans have increased their consumption of added sugar by 355 calories a day—the equivalent of 22 teaspoons! (*Added sugar* means any sugar or sugary syrup added to food during processing or preparation.) It's staggering to think that so much extra sugar is being sneaked into our food, and that the amount is soaring every year. And all that extra sugar is causing a lot of extra disease.

The increased intake, the AHA said, is linked to an increased risk of…

- High blood pressure

- High triglycerides (a blood fat that can damage arteries)

- Low levels of good HDL cholesterol

- Excessive weight

The statement from the AHA included these guidelines: Women shouldn't consume more than 100 calories of added sugar a day (six teaspoons, or two-thirds of a 12-ounce can of soda). Men shouldn't consume more than 150 calories (nine teaspoons, or a sip or so more than one can of soda).

Well, good luck with that, ladies and gentlemen—because reducing your intake of sugar and other refined carbohydrates is just as hard as quitting smoking, stopping drinking, kicking heroin or freeing yourself from any other tenacious *addiction.*

Are you addicted to refined carbs?

"Eating too much sugar is an addiction," said Dr. Teitelbaum. "Sugar gives you an initial high, you crash several hours later, and this leaves you wanting more sugar. If you crave sugar, telling you to cut your intake is like telling an addict to stop taking a drug." And Dr. Teitelbaum isn't the only MD who thinks sugar is addictive.

"Chips, cookies, ice cream and soda can become as addictive as any drug," I was told by Mark Hyman, MD, who also enumerated the ways in which processed foods—and their typical load of refined carbs—are addictive…

- Sugar, he says, stimulates the brain's pleasure or reward centers—just like addictive drugs.

- Foods rich in refined carbs also stimulate the body's internal opioids—biochemicals similar to morphine.

- And just like alcohol or heroin, you develop a *tolerance* for processed foods loaded with refined carbs—you need more and more to provide the same level of satisfaction. Eventually, you eat a lot refined carbs not to feel *better*, but just to feel *normal.*

- You experience "withdrawal" when you try to go cold turkey and completely give up the stuff you're addicted to.

And so when you try to "just say no" to refined carbs, you can't, even though you know they're no good for you—just the same way an alcoholic can't say no to a shot of whiskey and a heroin addict keeps shooting up.

A low-carb lifetime: Impossible, for most of us

Of course, you could try to kick your carb addiction by going on one of the many popular low-carb diets, like Atkins or South Beach. And many people do go on those diets. For a while.

But in a study of weight-loss diets, conducted by researchers at the Tufts-New England Medical Center and published in the *Journal of the American Medical Association*, 47% of the people on the Atkins diet dropped out. [3]

I'm guessing you don't need the results of a scientific study to convince you that the low-carb lifestyle isn't sustainable. After all, how many people do you know who maintain a low-carb diet? Who eat little or no sugar and white flour? Do you know *anybody* who has successfully limited their refined carbs day after day and year after year? Have you tried a low-carb diet—and stuck with it? The answer is probably no.

Here is the reality of your situation: You either can't or won't sustain the low-carb intake that can protect you from (or help you control) blood sugar problems, heart disease and being overweight. (That's certainly true for most of the clients in my health coaching practice. They're not "bad" people—they're just human beings who enjoy yummy, high-carb food! Congratulations if you're one of the exceptions!)

That's the bad news. Here's the good news—no, the *astounding* news:

You can dramatically cut back on refined carbs—*without* going on a low-carb diet.

That assertion is so amazing, I'll repeat it, in a slightly different way: You can cut your intake of carbs—*without* eating fewer carbs.

How is that possible? Simple:

All you have to do is take a safe and effective, all-natural supplement that *blocks* the absorption of carbohydrates in the digestive tract—a supplement called a carb-blocker. In other words, you *can* have your cake and eat it too! Let me show you how…

The doctor who takes his own medicine: Carb-blockers

When I want to find out the latest about carb-blockers, I always call Harry Preuss, MD, CNS (certified nutrition specialist). Dr. Preuss is a professor of physiology, medicine and pathology at Georgetown University Medical Center, and was my co-author on *The Natural Fat-Loss Pharmacy*, a book about supplements for weight loss—a book that included a chapter on carb-blockers.

Dr. Preuss has conducted several scientific studies on carb-blockers that have been published in the *Nutrition Journal*, the *International Journal of Medical Sciences* and *The Journal of Applied Research*.

And he summarized all of the research on carb-blockers in a scientific review paper titled "Bean Amylase Inhibitor and Other Carbohydrate Absorption Blockers: Effects on Diabesity and General Health," published in the *Journal of the American College of Nutrition*. [4]

I asked Dr. Preuss to sum up his best understanding about carb blockers for the readers of this Special Report—and to offer his best recommendations for daily intake. But first, I asked him if he uses carb-blockers himself.

"Well, as you know Bill, I *adore* Italian food—including pasta," he said. "So, whenever I go out to eat a big Italian dinner, I take along a couple of carb-blocker supplements to take before the meal. It blocks carbohydrate calories from being absorbed, and helps keep my blood sugar steady. As a man in his sixties who watches his weight and wants to prevent diabetes and heart disease, both those benefits are important to me."

Blocking the enzyme that breaks down carbs

Carb-blockers, Dr. Preuss explained, are extracts of white kidney beans (*phaseolus vulgaris*). They work by blocking the action of *alpha amylase*, a digestive enzyme secreted by the pancreas that breaks down carbs in the saliva and the small intestine—so fewer carbs are broken down and absorbed.

Carb-blockers were discovered in the 1950s. Early versions were sold over-the-counter in the early 1980s, but didn't work very well. Improved in the late 1980s, the new, effective generation of carb-blockers has been studied extensively in the last two decades.

Carb-blockers mainly work on *starchy* foods, like bread, cake, cookies, chips, pasta, rice and potatoes. But, says Dr. Preuss, his research shows they can also block sugar (sucrose) absorption.

Let's take a closer look at some of the research showing carb-blockers can help you balance blood sugar and shed pounds—some of it conducted by Dr. Preuss, and some by other researchers in the U.S. and around the world.

Science-proven results

66% less carb absorption. In a 2009 study, scientists at the University of Scranton fed 11 people sliced white bread—with and without a dose of 1,500 milligrams (mg) of carb blockers. Those taking the supplement absorbed 66% fewer carbs! [5]

In a similar study conducted by Dr. Preuss and his colleagues, a big dose of carb-blocker reduced the *glycemic index* (GI) of white bread by 34%. [6] (The GI is a scientific measurement of how much a carb-containing food increases blood sugar—with low GI foods like beans and vegetables linked to the prevention and control of diabetes, obesity and heart disease.)

Important: The scientists in both studies used Phase 2 carb blocker, manufactured by Pharmachem, and the main ingredient in many carb-blocking supplements. As a health coach, it's the carb blocker I recommend to my clients, because it's the best-studied.

Big drop in blood sugar. In a two-month study of 39 overweight people, those taking a carb-blocker with their meals had a drop in blood sugar of 22 mg/dl—five times greater than those on the placebo! [7] They also experienced much less hunger between meals and lost twice as much weight.

"I treat overweight patients with a low-calorie diet, advice on physical activity—and a carb-blocker containing supplement," I was told by Professor Mariangela Rondanelli, the study's lead author.

Eight times more weight loss. Dr. Preuss and his colleagues (including the dermatologist and bestselling author, Nicholas Perricone, MD) conducted a one-month study on carb-blockers in Italy. (What better place to test a carb-blocker than the Land of Pasta?). Sixty overweight but healthy people ate a 2,200-calorie diet that included lots of carbs at one meal—and took either a 450-mg carb blocker (Phase 2) or a placebo (a fake, lookalike pill) with the carb-rich meal. Those taking the carb blocker lost 6.5 pounds—compared to less than a pound for people taking a placebo. [8]

Triple the drop in triglycerides. Once eaten, refined carbohydrates can turn into *triglycerides*—a potentially deadly fat. "Elevated triglycerides are very common in people who have diabetes and are obese—and increase your risk of heart attack threefold," I was told by Steven Joyal, MD, author of *What Your Doctor May Not Tell You About Diabetes*. Carb blockers can tame triglycerides, too…

In a study of 50 obese people conducted by researchers at UCLA, those who took a 1,500 mg carb-blocker (Phase 2) twice a day with meals had a 26% drop in triglycerides—triple the drop in people taking a placebo. [9]

"If you're looking for a supplement to accelerate the benefits of a good diet and regular exercise, a carb-blocker can be helpful," I was told by Jay Udani, MD, the study's lead researcher.

Three success stories

Let's switch from the rarified air of scientific studies to the real-world struggles of everyday people. Do carb-blockers work for them? Definitely!

"I lowered my blood sugar." "When I reached my mid-50s, I had become a borderline diabetic, and my doctor said I had to do something," said Terry V., from New York. "I tried a low-carb diet, but found it was tough to stick to. Then I discovered a dietary supplement containing a carb-blocker. Now, when I eat carbs, I also take a couple of pills. Well, I have lowered my blood sugar…and lost 76 pounds…and improved my cholesterol levels. (In fact, my doctor recently took me off my cholesterol-lowering drug.) I don't eat carbs unless I take the carb-blocker."

"I lost three to four pounds a week." "I was 35-years-old, 5'2" tall and weighed 168 pounds," said Carla C., from Canada. "I had tried weight loss supplements but never had any success. I work as a Customer Service Manager for a Wal-Mart in Ontario, saw a carb-blocker on the shelves, and decided to give it a try. After taking it for a week I weighed myself—and thought my scale must have broken, because I had lost three pounds. I can't believe losing weight is this easy—I just take the carb-blocker before eating foods with lots of carbohydrates. As time went on, my appetite has decreased, I've continued to lose three to four pounds a week—and I've reached my goal weight of 116 pounds! I told several friends from work and many customers about carb-blockers—and they've had success with weight loss, too."

"I was hypersensitive to carbs." "I've had problems with controlling my blood sugar levels for 30 years," said Kathy A., from California. "Combined with a tendency to overeat, it's been very difficult to achieve and maintain an optimum weight. I started taking a carb-blocker supplement, hoping it would help me with my blood sugar. Amazingly, it did! I am hypersensitive to carbs, but the carb-blocker evened out my blood sugar levels. I've also lost a few pounds, and my weight loss goal is within reach. I'm hooked!"

The right dose, the right supplement

In writing this chapter, I talked to many researchers, doctors and other experts, asking them to recommend the *best* carb-blocker, at the *right* dose. Here's what they said…

A higher dose is more effective. In the many studies on carb-blockers, the dose has ranged from 100 to 1,000 mg per meal. What level works best?

Higher doses of carb-blocker are always better, because the supplement works by blocking the alpha-amylase enzyme that breaks down refined carbohydrates, said Dr. Udani. In other words, the more carb-blocker you take, the more carbs you block. That means the higher dose—1,000 mg per meal—is the ideal dose.

Take the supplement right before you eat. When Dr. Preuss uses a carb-blocker, he takes it about 15 minutes before the meal. "I think studies have shown that's the best timing," he told me.

Laura Garett, RD, CDE, a registered dietician and certified diabetes educator, always advises clients to take 1,000 mg either *right before* a high-carb meal, or *with the meal*—opening two, 500 mg capsules and sprinkling the (tasteless) powder on the carbs. "That way, you start the inhibition of the amylase enzyme right in the mouth," she told me.

Use the science-proven carb-blocker. Most of the scientific studies on carb-blockers have used Phase 2, from Pharmachem. Examples of supplements with Phase 2 include: Carb Neutralizer, from Hyperion Natural Solutions; Carb-Intercept with Phase 2 from Natrol; Phase 2 Starch Neutralizer from Swanson; and Phase 2 Starch Neutralizer from Now.

One other important fact to know about Phase 2: In 2006, the FDA wrote a letter to Pharmachem, approving the use of these two claims for the ingredient:

- "May reduce the enzymatic digestion of dietary starches."

- "May assist in weight control when used in conjunction with a sensible diet and exercise program."

Phase 2 is *the only* over-the-counter nutritional ingredient FDA-approved to make these two claims.

Don't fret about safety. "I don't think there are any safety issues with carb-blockers," said Dr. Preuss. "Big doses are safe in animals. There are no side effects in clinical studies. And there has been a decade of problem-free use in the marketplace.

Caution: If you are taking anti-diabetes medication, tell your doctor you're taking the supplement. Carb-blockers work so well that a person with diabetes may need less glucose-controlling medication, said Dr. Udani. "If you have diabetes and are on medication, tell your doctor you're taking the supplement," he advised. (That same advice goes for *every* supplement I discuss in *Defeat High Blood Sugar — Naturally!*)

Special advice for those with diabetes

"Ideally, a person with diabetes will limit their carbohydrate intake—and completely eliminate their intake of refined sugar," said Garett. "But many of my clients tell me, 'I can't stop eating bread,' or 'I can't stop eating pasta.' For those people, carb-blockers are an important tool—for example, they can eat 2 cups of cooked pasta and, by taking a carb-blocker at the same time, it's as if they only ate 1 cup.

"The person with diabetes doesn't need to use a carb-blocker if they're having a chicken salad with three croutons. But for a meal or other occasion that includes starchy food—rice, potatoes, noodles, pasta, cake, bread, pretzels and the like—carb-blockers can be a smart and useful supplement."

"Carb-blockers aren't a miracle," adds Dr. Preuss. "You can't eat a pint of ice cream and take a carb-blocker and expect your blood sugar and weight to be A-okay. Carb-blockers are an *aid* to a balanced diet. They give you a little more dietary leeway, so that you don't have to stick to an excessively low-carb diet in order to control your blood sugar and lose weight."

Sugar-blockers work, too

As you learned in this chapter, the white kidney bean extract found in carb-blockers stops the action of *alpha amylase*, the enzyme that breaks down starch so it can be absorbed and digested.

Well, another compound—L-arabinose—stops or slows the action of the digestive enzyme *sucrase*, which breaks down sugar in the intestines. In other words, it's a *sugar-blocker*. And it blocks like an NFL lineman.

Newest finding: In a study conducted by Dr. Preuss and his colleagues, 50 adults who didn't have diabetes drank a big glass of sugar water and had their blood sugar and insulin levels measured—first, when they just drank the sugar water; next, when they drank the sugar water *and* took a sugar-blocker with 1,000 mg of L-arabinose.

In the 90-minute period after drinking the sugar water, the sugar-blocker reduced blood sugar by an average of 24% and insulin by an average of 28%.

"The data support the hypothesis that l-arabinose worked by blocking sucrose absorption," wrote the researchers in *Nutrition Journal.* [10]

L-arabinose is available from Pharmachem as the ingredient Phase 3—an ingredient found in Carb Neutralizer from Hyperion Natural Solutions, and in the supplement Optimized Irvingia with Phase 3 Calorie Control, from LifeExtension. (*Irvingia gabonensis* is a plant from West Africa. A 2009 study in *Lipids in Health and Disease* found that an extract from its seeds aided weight loss and lowered total cholesterol, bad LDL cholesterol and blood sugar levels. [11])

"Using a carb-blocker *and* a sugar-blocker at the same time might be even more effective in controlling blood sugar and insulin levels than using either supplement alone," Dr. Preuss told me.

The newest carb-blocker on the block: transglucosidase

As you'll read in the next chapter, on the super-fiber supplement PGX, adding fiber to a meal is one of the best ways to blunt the carb-caused, post-meal spikes in blood sugar that injure your arteries and ruin your health.

But what if you could take a supplement that magically turns glucose-spiking starch *into* fiber? Sounds like a pipedream, right?

Not so, say a team of digestive specialists from a medical school in Japan. They've been conducting studies on *transglucosidase* (TG), an enzyme that converts starches into *oligosaccharides,* a component of fiber. Here are some of the astounding results…

White rice is no match for transglucosidase. When the scientists gave starchy meals of rice balls *and* a transglucosidase supplement to people with pre-diabetes, they had lower post-meal levels of both glucose and insulin. "These results suggest that transglucosidase may be useful for preventing the progression of type 2 diabetes," wrote the researchers in the *Journal of Clinical Biochemistry and Nutrition.* [12]

Lowering blood sugar and insulin. In another study, the researchers divided people with diabetes into two groups: one group took a transglucosidase supplement every day and the other didn't. After three months, those taking the enzyme had bigger drops in A1C and insulin. They also had lower LDL, triglycerides and body fat. [13]

More friendly bacteria, lower blood sugar—with transglucosidase. Oligosaccharides are *prebiotics*—the nourishment for *probiotics,* health-giving bacteria in your gut. And as you'll read in Chapter 7, the latest research shows that probiotics can help normalize blood sugar.

Sure enough, the Japanese researchers found that 60 people with diabetes who took a daily transglucosidase supplement for three months had more probiotics in their intestines—and better blood sugar and weight control than people not taking the supplement. [14]

If you want to try a transglucosidase supplement, I suggest GlycemiaPro Transglucosidase, from LifeExtension, a trustworthy brand. As with any other carb-blocker, take it right before or with a high-carb meal. Follow the dosage recommendation on the label.

Anti-diabetes secrets in the next chapter...

- Scientists call controlling this mealtime metabolic event "the most important" factor in long-term blood sugar control. And you *can* control it—with PGX, the super-supplement featured in the next chapter.

- Feeling mentally fuzzy after meals? Here's how to prevent a post-meal drop in concentration and memory.

- Discover the mealtime "magic wand" that instantly turns bad carbs like white rice into the equivalent of good carbs like brown rice. (Yes, it's that *simple*. And that powerful.)

- The natural diabetes remedy one delighted user calls "better than metformin."

EXPERTS AND CONTRIBUTORS:

Laura Garett, RD, CDE, is a registered dietician, certified diabetes educator and founder of Realtime Nutrition, Inc, which provides marketing and communications services for food companies and PR and marketing agencies.
Website: www.realtime-nutrition.com.

Frank Hu, MD, PhD, is a professor of nutrition and epidemiology at the Harvard School of Public Health.

Mark Hyman, MD, was co-medical director of Canyon Ranch for almost 10 years and is now the chairman of the Institute for Functional Medicine and founder and medical director of the UltraWellness Center. He is the *New York Times* bestselling author of *UltraMetabolism, The UltraMind Solution*, and the *UltraSimple Diet*.
Websites: www.drhyman.com, www.bloodsugarsolution.com
Facebook: facebook.com/drmarkhyman
Twitter: @markhymanmd

Richard J. Johnson, MD, is a professor of medicine at the University of Colorado, Denver, and author of *The Sugar Fix: The High-Fructose Fallout That Is Making You Fat And Sick.*

Steven V. Joyal, MD, is the vice president of Scientific Affairs and Medical Development of the Life Extension Foundation, and author of *What Your Doctor May Not Tell You About Diabetes: An Innovative Program to Prevent, Treat, and Beat This Controllable Disease.*

Harry Preuss, MD, CNS, is a professor of physiology, medicine and pathology at Georgetown University Medical Center, and author of more than 350 medical papers. He is also a Certified Nutrition Specialist (CNS) and past president of the American College of Nutrition. He is the co-author of *The Natural Fat-Loss Pharmacy.*

Mariangela Rondanelli, MD, is a Professor of Medicine in the Department of Applied Health Sciences in the Section of Human Nutrition and Dietetics at the University of Pavia in Italy.

Jacob Teitelbaum, MD, is a board certified internist and Medical Director of the national Fibromyalgia and Fatigue Centers and Chronicity. He is author of the popular free iPhone application *Cures A-Z*, and author of the bestselling book *From Fatigued to Fantastic!*, as well as *Pain Free 1-2-3* (McGraw-Hill), *Three Steps to Happiness: Healing Through Joy* and *Beat Sugar Addiction NOW!*. His newest book is *Real Cause, Real Cure.*
Website: www.endfatigue.com

Jay Udani, MD, is an assistant clinical professor at UCLA School of Medicine, Medical Director of the Integrative Medicine Program at Northridge Hospital in Northridge, California, and an adjunct professor in the research division of Southern California University of Health Sciences.

REFERENCES:

1. Malik VS, et al. Sugar-sweetened beverages and risk of metabolic syndrome and type 2 diabetes: a meta-analysis. *Diabetes Care.* 2010 Nov;33(11):2477-83.

2. Malik VS, et al. Sweeteners and Risk of Obesity and Type 2 Diabetes: The Role of Sugar-Sweetened Beverages. *Current Diabetes Reports.* 2012 Jan 31.2012 Jan 31. [Epub ahead of print]

3. Dansinger ML, et al. Comparison of the Atkins, Ornish, Weight Watchers, and Zone diets for weight loss and heart disease risk reduction: a randomized trial. *Journal of the American Medical Association.* 2005 Jan 5;293(1):43-53.

4. Preuss, HG. Bean Amylase Inhibitor and Other Carbohydrate Absorption Blockers: Effects on Diabesity and General Health. *Journal of the American College of Nutrition*, Vol. 28, No., 3, 266-276 (2009)

5. Vinson JA, et al. Investigation of an amylase inhibitor on human glucose absorption after starch consumption. *Open Nutraceuticals Journal*, 2:88-91, 2009.

6. Udani, JK, et al. Lowering the glycemic index of white bread using a white bean extract. *Nutrition Journal*, Oct 28;8:52.

7. Rondanelli M, et al. Appetite Control and Glycaemia Reduction in Overweight Subjects treated with a Combination of Two Highly Standardized Extracts from Phaseolus vulgaris and Cynara scolymus. *Phytotherapy Research.* 2011 Feb 10. doi: 10.1002/ptr.3425.

8. Celleno L, et al. Effect of a dietary supplement containing standardized *Phaseolus vulgaris* extract on the body composition of overweight men and women. *International Journal of Medical Sciences*, 4:45-52, 2007.

9. Udani, J, et al. Blocking carbohydrate absorption and weight loss: a clinical trial using Phase 2 brand proprietary fractionated white bean extract. *Alternative Medicine Review*, 9:63-69, 2004.

10. Kaats, GR, et al. A combination of l-arabinose and chromium lowers circulating glucose and insulin levels after an acute oral sucrose challenge. *Nutrition Journal*, 2011, May 6;10(1):42.

11. Ngondi JL, et al. IGOB131, a novel seed extract of the West African plant Irvingia gabonensis, significantly reduces body weight and improves metabolic parameters in overweight humans in a randomized double-blind placebo controlled investigation. *Lipids in Health and Disease*, 2009 Mar 2;8:7.

12. Sasaki M, et al. A Novel Strategy in Production of Oligosaccharides in Digestive Tract: Prevention of Postprandial Hyperglycemia and Hyperinsulinemia. *Journal of Clinical Biochemistry and Nutrition*, 41, 191-96, November 2007.

13. Sasaki M, et al. Effects of transglucosidase on diabetes, cardiovascular risk factors and hepatic biomarkers in patients with type 2 diabetes: a 12-week, randomized, double-blind, placebo-controlled trial. *Diabetes, Obesity and Metabolism*, 2012 Apr;14(4):379-82.

14. Sasaki M, et al. Transglucosidase improves the gut microbiota profile of type 2 diabetes mellitus patients: a randomized double-blind, placebo-controlled study. *BMC Gastroenterology*, 2013 May 8;13:81.

Chapter 5

PGX

Super-fiber for post-meal blood sugar control

The riskiest time of day is the two hours right after a big meal, when your body turns food into fuel.

Scientists have dubbed this post-meal period *postprandial*. And it's a well-established scientific fact that preventing *postprandial hyperglycemia*—when a meal loaded with carbs morphs into a flood of circulating blood sugar—is a must for controlling both diabetes and heart disease (the deadly illness that follows diabetes like its shadow).

I'll like to introduce you to PGX, the best supplement for preventing post-meal glucose spikes.

As you'll learn in the rest of the chapter, PGX has helped folks with blood sugar problems…cut post-meal blood sugar spikes by 50%….shed pounds fast (one doctor reports a patient lost 40 pounds *just* by taking PGX)…reverse prediabetes…stop taking diabetes medications, as PGX brought their blood sugar under control….and lower artery-clogging LDL cholesterol.

Here's what one person with diabetes said about the supplement:

"I was diagnosed with diabetes eight months ago," said JW. "I was told I had to take six different medications and 66 units of insulin every day, which I did—when I could afford it. Then I found out about PGX and started taking it. I checked my A1C blood sugar for 6 weeks while on PGX and it was always between 5 and 8—and I lost 35 pounds. So I haven't done any pills or insulin for about four months. And my blood sugar is where it's supposed to be."

PGX is extraordinary. And, as I mentioned a moment ago, the main reason it's so powerful is because it prevents post-meal glucose spikes. Studies show that preventing postprandial hyperglycemia can help…

- **Prevent diabetes.** Post-meal spikes in blood sugar are a "major determinant" of A1C, the standard measurement of long-term blood sugar control, declared a scientific paper in *Diabetes*. [1] In other words, if you can stop those post-meal spikes, you'll basically get your blood sugar under control.

- **Manage prediabetes so it doesn't become diabetes.** Keeping post-meal glucose spikes under control reduces the risk of prediabetes advancing to diabetes by 36%, reported a study in the prestigious medical journal *Lancet*. [2]

- **Manage diabetes so it doesn't advance.** Several studies show that the post-meal glucose level is "the most important" factor in long-term blood sugar control in people with diabetes, according to a scientific paper in *Diabetes Care* on postprandial glucose levels. [3]

- **Prevent diabetic complications,** like neuropathy, leg ulcers and vision loss. "Evidence accumulates that postprandial excursions [spikes] of blood glucose may be involved in the development of diabetes complications," declared a scientific paper in *Diabetes*. [1]

- **Prevent weight problems.** One obesity researcher I talked to (who I'll introduce later in the chapter) found that *everybody* who gains weight has one thing in common: poor, post-meal blood sugar control. "Almost every person with a weight problem has abnormal spikes and drops in glucose levels," he told me. "These 'excursions' are the key—and neglected—factor behind the inability to lose weight and keep it off."

- **Prevent memory loss, poor concentration and dementia.** Diabetes quadruples the risk for Alzheimer's disease, with some researchers now calling Alzheimer's "Type 3 Diabetes." Well, in a scientific paper titled "Impact of postprandial glycaemia on health and prevention of disease," published in *Obesity Reviews* in 2012, the authors theorized that the inflammation and cell-damaging free radicals triggered by glucose spikes not only hurt the heart—they also hurt the brain. And a brain-bashing rush of glucose not only sets you up for problems in the future. Studies show that it also befuddles your brain *immediately,* worsening everyday memory and concentration. [4]

- **Prevent heart attacks and strokes (cardiovascular disease),** the events that actually kill most people with diabetes. Control of post-meal glucose levels lowers the risk of high blood pressure by 34% and the risk of heart attack and stroke by 49%, reported a study in the *Journal of the American Medical Association*. [5]

In fact, your levels of postprandial glucose are a *better predictor* of whether or not you'll die of heart disease than your level of fasting glucose (wrongly considered by many to be the best indicator of the severity of diabetes)—and that's true for folks with and without diabetes. [6]

Why are glucose spikes so deadly?

Top experts say the best blood glucose level during the two hours after a meal is under 140. But why are higher levels so damaging? Because they…

Spark the oxidation of LDL cholesterol, a process that slathers on the plaque.

Trigger increases in artery-clogging cholesterol and triglycerides.

Damage artery linings (endothelium), making them harder, less flexible, and more prone to plaque buildup.

Thicken blood, making it more likely to clot and block an artery.

Boost inflammatory factors that drive heart disease.

Trigger the production of free radicals, unstable molecules that damage cells—including arterial cells.

The bottom line about glucose spikes and your heart: Multiple studies, involving thousands of people with diabetes, prove that a sharp rise in post-meal blood sugar damages arteries, setting you up for a heart attack or stroke.

A 2012 scientific paper on the topic—"Impact of postprandial glycaemia on health and prevention of disease"—summarizes all those studies:

"Evidence indicates that abnormal elevations in glycemia after a meal…are linked with increased risk of morbidity [poor health] and mortality [death] due to cardiovascular disease in individuals with or without type 2 diabetes." [4]

In other words, a dietary spike of glucose drives a spike into your heart—whether you have prediabetes, diabetes, or don't have diabetes at all.

Enough said. Now let's find out how to *fix* the problem. Fortunately, the solution couldn't be simpler…

Blunting the spike

There's an incredibly easy way to blunt post-meal spikes of blood sugar: right before you eat, take a supplement of the super-fiber PGX (PolyGlycopleX).

This unique fiber supplement was formulated by Michael Lyon, MD, medical director of the Canadian Centre for Functional Medicine in British Columbia, and author of several books, including *How to Prevent and Treat Diabetes with Natural Medicine* and *Hunger-Free Forever*, both of which feature PGX.

Dr. Lyon also has co-authored most of the scientific studies proving the unique efficacy of PGX. (There are more than a dozen.)

I'm also happy to say that Dr. Lyon and I are on a first-name basis. I've interviewed him several times about PGX, and we've talked about someday writing a book together that features the supplement.

But I'm going to introduce you to a few other folks before you hear more from Michael—folks who have benefitted from his super-fiber formulation…folks who were so impressed by the health effects of PGX that they felt compelled to write the manufacturer (Natural Factors) to let the company know about their balanced blood sugar, weight loss and good health. I think it's best to share these testimonials first, because you'll be even more excited to read the details about PGX.

PGX success stories

Reduced insulin. "I have been diabetic for 26 years," said PK. "Now, with PGX, <u>I have been able to reduce my insulin</u>—and I have lost weight!"

Blood sugar no longer spikes. "I'm taking two caps of PGX Daily [a nutritional supplement] with each meal and I think it's amazing," said RR. "<u>I've found my blood sugar no longer spikes and plummets like it used to</u>."

Off medication. "I am a health practitioner and I think PGX is a great product," said GS. "My husband, who is a diabetic, was on the medication metformin. I was able to keep a close watch on his blood sugar levels—and now <u>he is completely off his medication</u>. And he lost 22 pounds. He tried the meal replacements but there was too much sugar in them and they spiked his blood sugar levels. But just using the PGX capsule has really helped him. We have told several other people with diabetes about PGX."

"Awesome." "I have used PGX for about three months, and it is *awesome*," said RG. "I have recommended it to at least four people who are now taking it and really happy with the results—<u>they've all improved their blood sugar levels and lost weight</u>."

Reversing prediabetes. "Before starting PGX, I was prediabetic," said LC. "<u>Three weeks after starting it, my blood sugar was normalized</u>. And over the past several years I have lost 70 pounds!"

"Better than metformin." "I was told I was a type 2 diabetic," said MP. "I went on metformin for more than a year, and also took cholesterol medication. But even with all my medications, my glycemic level was going up, along with the dosage. I also went from 250 to 272 pounds. Then I heard about PGX and figured, why not. I started to take three to four pills per meal, without exception—and I even took a pill with each snack! <u>The results were extraordinary.</u> <u>My glycemic level is back down to normal, between 5.5 to 6.0</u>—and I feel very good now that my blood sugar is under control. And I have lost 15 pounds in the last 2 months. This is the best natural product that I have ever used in my life—it is better than metformin and cholesterol medication."

The discovery of PGX

Now that you've read about the amazing effectiveness of PGX in controlling and reversing blood sugar problems and losing weight, you're probably eager to hear about *what* it is and *how* to use it. Let's begin *before* the beginning…

Before the invention of PGX, scientists already understood that *soluble fiber* (found in foods like beans, oats, apples, carrots and psyllium seeds) created a thick, slow-moving slurry in the stomach and small intestine—a slurry that slows the rate at which carbohydrates turn into glucose. (This rate is called the *Glycemic Index*, or GI—the faster the absorption of carbohydrates, the higher the GI. White bread has a GI of 100; broccoli, 15.)

Scientists also knew the thicker or more *viscous* the soluble fiber, the better it was at slowing the digestion of carbs and keeping blood sugar levels steady.

But since most of us don't eat beans, oats, apples and carrots on a regular basis, scientists tried to create a highly viscous, soluble fiber *supplement*—a fiber-rich powder, flake or granule that could be added to food. But there were a couple of problems with those supplements.

They *tasted* terrible.

They *felt* terrible in the mouth, forming a gooey paste.

They *looked* terrible. Stirred into a glass of water, they immediately formed an unappealing glop.

They *didn't work* terribly well. The supplements didn't have much digestive staying-power: they were viscous in the glass, but not in the stomach and small intestines.

Surveying this field of failed fiber, Dr. Lyon set out to create the perfect soluble fiber supplement.

"We tested many fiber blends and they became thick very quickly," he told me. "They glued up in the teeth and mouth, and tasted awful."

"Also, they didn't have any stability," he continued. "They were thick in the glass, but they didn't stay thick in the intestinal tract."

So Dr. Lyon and his colleagues started processing the fibers.

They preheated them. They applied pressure to them. They did everything they could think of to produce a fiber that was highly thick or viscous…pleasant to consume…and stayed viscous in the gut. And after trying more than *one thousand* variations, they finally succeeded—big time.

They produced the super-fiber PGX: a specially processed combination of three viscous fibers: konjac powder, sodium alginate and xanthan gum.

Why a *super*-fiber? Because it's *super*ior to all others

PGX can't leap tall buildings in a single bound—but it did leapfrog all other fibers in its power to solve the problem of post-meal glucose spikes. PGX…

- **had 3 to 5 times more viscosity than any other soluble fiber.**

- **had delayed viscosity**—sprinkled on food or mixed with juice or water, it didn't immediately thicken, so it was palatable.

- **stayed viscous in the small intestine.**

- **lowered the GI of high GI foods by up to 60%**—an effect never before produced by any other fiber. (Glycemic index or GI is a measure of how fast carbs turn into blood sugar after you swallow them.)

It was found that PGX lowers a food's glycemic index remarkably – turning low-fiber carbs into high-fiber carbs that turn into blood sugar at a slower rate. For example, white bread baked with PGX has a *lower* GI than whole-wheat bread. White rice with PGX sprinkled on it has a lower GI than brown rice. Which makes PGX a little bit like a mealtime magic wand—you "wave" it over food and bad carbs change into good carbs!

"There is nothing else like PGX," Dr. Lyon told me—"no other fiber that consistently lowers the GI of whatever food you eat it with."

But the good news doesn't end there.

Solving post-meal problems—with PGX

Dr. Lyon and his colleagues (including Jenny Brand-Miller, PhD, an acknowledged world-class expert in the GI Index, and co-author of *The New Glucose Revolution*) have conducted three studies on PGX and post-prandial glycemia, reporting their findings in the *European Journal of Clinical Nutrition*. [7]

In the studies, they gave people PGX as either a nutritional supplement (a soft gel capsule) or a granulated powder dissolved in water. The participants took PGX right before, with and/or after meals. The results were spectacular.

50% reduction in blood sugar spikes following a meal (postprandial hyperglycemia). Taken right before the meal, the powdered supplement cut post-meal blood sugar levels *in half*—a huge decrease. And the more PGX the participants took, the lower their post-meal blood sugar levels.

The powdered form of the fiber was effective at reducing glucose levels in the hours after a meal.

And the PGX capsule just kept on working—*taken at dinner, the nutritional supplement lowered glucose levels after the next morning's breakfast*! (Though not as much as PGX taken with a meal.)

"I recommend PGX wholeheartedly," Dr. Brand told me. "It's a very simple, palatable and effective way to lower blood glucose levels after a meal—and it's superior to every other type of fiber." (The best way to use PGX for lower blood sugar levels is along with a low-GI, high-protein diet, she added.)

In another study, Dr. Lyon and his colleagues wanted to find out if PGX could control post-meal glucose levels after study participants ate various foods and meals, including cornflakes, rice, strawberry yogurt, granola, white bread, and a frozen turkey dinner. No matter the food, PGX did the job.

"Sprinkling or incorporation of PGX into a variety of different foods is highly effective in reducing postprandial glycemia," concluded the researchers in *Nutrition Journal*. [8]

And reducing post-meal blood sugar spikes with PGX not only improves your health—it might add years to your life.

"These postprandial blood sugar surges turn on a storm of free radicals that cause massive oxidative stress and an inflammatory cascade," Michael Lyon, MD, told me. "Regardless of whether you lose weight or not, regardless of whether you're diabetic or not, stopping those surges with PGX is likely to add years to your life."

PGXtraordinary, I'd say.

"Profound effects on glucose, insulin and A1C"

And so would Mark Hyman, MD, chairman of the Institute for Functional Medicine, and founder and medical director of the UltraWellness Center in Lennox, Massachusetts.

"This super fiber has *profound* effects on glucose, insulin and A1C," he told me. "It can lower your blood sugar after a meal by 50%, your overall blood sugar levels by 23%, and your bad LDL cholesterol by 20%.

"And by reducing the absorption of sugar and fats in the bloodstream, it helps to not only control blood sugar and cholesterol, but also helps control appetite, speeding weight loss.

"I recommend taking it before meals with a glass of water to help control diabetes and obesity. I have had patients lose up to 40 pounds—just by using this super fiber."

Dr. Hyman is making a key point: When you take PGX before a meal, you feel fuller sooner…and you don't feel hungry afterwards…because your blood sugar is stable. In other words, you don't *want to overeat* at the meal or after the meal—the ideal condition for losing weight and keeping it off.

More standout studies on PGX

There are several other superb studies on PGX, conducted by Dr. Lyon and his colleagues.

A fiber your tummy can love. Some people don't like to use fiber supplements because they can cause bloating, gas and other forms of digestive discomfort. But in a study in *Nutrition Journal*, involving 54 healthy folks aged 18 to 55, Dr. Lyon found that taking 10 grams a day (5 with lunch and 5 with dinner) didn't produce any excess gas or bloating. And while those who took the fiber didn't have high blood sugar to correct, they *still* had hefty drops in bad LDL and total cholesterol. "PGX is well-tolerated as part of a regular diet," concluded the researchers. [9]

Reducing Glycemic Index by 30%. In a 2012 study in the *British Journal of Nutrition*, researchers found that a 5 gram dose of PGX reduced the glycemic index of six, high-carb foods by an average of 30%—a whopping amount. [10]

Boosting PYY, the "satiety hormone." PYY (peptide YY) is a hormone that controls appetite, helping you feel less hungry. In a study of 54 people, those who took PGX for three weeks had a steady level of PYY—while those who didn't use the fiber saw a steady drop in the hormone. [11]

Losing 12 pounds in two weeks. Twenty-nine overweight people participated in a study of PGX, taking the supplement (5 grams in water) before meals, 2 to 3 times a day, for two weeks. They lost an average of 12.7 pounds, their waist size shrank by nearly 5 inches, and their percentage of body fat dropped by 2.4. They also had a 19% drop in total cholesterol and a 26% drop in LDL. [12]

How to Use PGX

Okay, now you know that taking PGX is a science-proven way to lower post-meal glucose—and plenty of folks have used it with great success to control blood sugar and lose weight. So how do *you* use it?

PGX is available as a nutritional supplement (soft gel capsule) and as granules that you either sprinkle on food or mix with water. Here are Dr. Lyon's recommendations about how to use those two forms…

Use PGX with a meal. Sprinkle 5 grams (a level teaspoon) of the granular form onto a moist food, such as rice or pasta…into a soup…into a sauce that you're adding to a food…into yogurt…or into a smoothie before you blend it.

"The granules are the most effective form for controlling blood sugar, and they're the most cost-effective, too," he said.

And don't worry about the taste.

"PGX really doesn't have any taste," Dr. Lyon said. "It takes on the flavor of whatever it's combined with."

The granules are sold either in bulk (a large container with a 5-gram scoop) or in individual, per-meal, 5-gram packets.

Important: If you add PGX to a food and let it sit for 20 minutes, it will congeal into an unpalatable gel. Eat your meal a few minutes after adding PGX.

Use PGX with a beverage. Sprinkle the granules into water immediately before the meal and drink the water, Dr. Lyon advised. "Or put PGX in a bottle of water, shake it and drink it," he added.

Important: In Dr. Lyon's studies, he tested taking the granules 30 minutes before a meal, 15 minutes before, and right before. Taking PGX at the *start* of a meal was most effective in keeping post-meal blood sugar under control.

Take PGX as a nutritional supplement. Take one or more soft gel capsules (PGX Daily) before a meal. In Dr. Lyon's research, the most effective doses were 3 grams, 4.5 grams and 6 grams. The capsules are available in 500 milligram and 750 milligram dosages. So you'd have to take four capsules to replicate Dr. Lyon's research. But remember: the granules—as a drink or sprinkled on a meal—are *far more effective* in regulating post-meal blood sugar than the capsules. They're also cheaper.

Finding PGX. The super-fiber is widely sold in retail stores in the US and Canada, and online. To find a store near you that sells PGX products, visit the website www.pgx.com. In the dropdown menu under "About PGX" go to "Where to Buy" and enter your address.

You can find the supplement in 500 mg and 750 mg capsules, and the granules in various flavors.

My suggestion: As a health coach, I always incorporate PGX into my clients' weight loss regimens. I suggest they use the granule form—which, as I said, is cheaper, and more effective than the capsules—in water, before every meal.

Anti-diabetes secrets in the next chapter...

- Discover why clinicians are calling berberine the "unknown miracle herb" and "the most powerful new diabetes remedy." (And why one doctor recommends you seriously consider switching *from* your diabetes drug *to* berberine, with your physician's okay.)

- High blood sugar plummeted from a skyrocketing 191 to a prediabetic 124—with berberine.

- The enthusiastic endorsement of a man who's had diabetes for 43 years—and finds berberine the BEST therapy he's ever used for controlling high blood sugar.

EXPERTS AND CONTRIBUTORS:

Dr. Jenny Brand-Miller is a Professor of Biochemistry in the School of Molecular Bioscience, Boden Institute of Obesity, Nutrition, Exercise & Eating Disorders, at the University of Sydney in Australia. She is the co-author of *The Low-GI Shopper's Guide to GI Values 2013*, *The New Glucose Revolution*, the *Low GI Diet* and many other books.
Website: www.glycemicindex.com

Mark Hyman, MD, was co-medical director of Canyon Ranch for almost ten years and is now the chairman of the Institute for Functional Medicine and founder and medical director of the UltraWellness Center. He is the *New York Times* bestselling author of *UltraMetabolism*, *The UltraMind Solution*, and *The UltraSimple Diet*.
Website: www.drhyman.com
Facebook: facebook.com/drmarkhyman
Twitter: @markhymanmd

Michael Lyon, MD, is the inventor of the super-fiber PolyGlycopleX, medical director of the Canadian Centre for Functional Medicine in British Columbia, and coauthor of *How to Prevent and Treat Diabetes with Natural Medicine* and *Hunger-Free Forever*.

REFERENCES:

1. Ceriello, A. Postprandial Hyperglycemia and Diabetes Complications. *Diabetes*, Vol. 54, January 2005.

2. Chiasson JL, et al. The STOP-NIDDM Trail Research Group: Acarbose for prevention of type 2 diabetes mellitus, *Lancet*, 359:2072-2077, 2002.

3. Ceriello A. Point: postprandial glucose levels are a clinically important treatment target. *Diabetes Care*, 2010, Aug; 33(8):1905-7.

4. Blaak, EE, et al. Impact of postprandial glycaemia on health and prevention of disease. *Obesity Reviews*, 13, 923-984, October 2012.

5. Chiasson, JL, et al. The STOP-NIDDM Trial Research Group: Acarbose treatment and the risk of cardiovascular disease and hypertension in patients with impaired glucose tolerance. *Journal of the American Medical Association*, 290:486-494, 2003.

6. Mah E, et al. Postprandial hyperglycemia on vascular endothelial function: mechanisms and consequences. *Nutrition Research*, 2012 Oct;32(10): 727-40.

7. Brand-Miller JC, et al. Effects of PGX, a novel functional fibre, on acute and delayed postprandial glycemia. *European Journal of Clinical Nutrition*, 2010 Dec;64(12):1488-93.

8. Jenkins, AL, et al. Reduction of postprandial glycemia by the novel viscous polysaccharide PGX, in a dose-dependent manner, independent of food form. *Journal of the American College of Nutrition,* 2010 Apr;29(2):92-8.

9. Carabin, IG, et al. Supplementation of the diet with the functional fiber PolyGlycoplex is well tolerated by healthy subjects in a clinical trial. *Nutrition Journal*, 2009 Feb 5;8:9.

10. Brand-Miller JC, et al. Effects of added PGX, a novel functional fibre, on the glycaemic index of starchy foods. *British Journal of Nutrition,* 2012 Jul;108(2):245-8.

11. Reimer, RA et al. Increased plasma PYY levels following supplementation with the functional fiber PolyGlycopleX in healthy adults. *European Journal of Clinical Nutrition*, 2010 Oct;64(10):1186-91.

12. Lyon, MR, The effect of a novel viscous polysaccharide along with lifestyle changes on short-term weight loss and associated risk factors in overweight and obese adults: an observational retrospective clinical program analysis. *Alternative Medicine Review,* 2010 Apr;15(1):68-75.

Chapter 6

Berberine

As effective as medication for diabetes—and a lot safer!

I'm a longtime fan (and friend) of Mark Stengler, ND, a naturopathic doctor in Encinitas, California, associate clinical professor at the National College of Naturopathic Medicine in Portland, Oregon, and author of 17 books, including the bestselling *Prescription for Natural Cures*.

I've interviewed Dr. Stengler many times for my books and articles on health, and can always count on him for balanced, science-backed and effective recommendations about natural remedies for everyday and serious health conditions.

So it was a no-brainer to call him while writing *Defeat High Blood Sugar – Naturally!*—and ask if there were any natural cures he was particularly excited about.

He didn't hesitate for a second.

"The most powerful new diabetes remedy is *berberine*, an herbal extract," he told me.

What's so special about berberine, I asked?

"Research shows that it can control diabetes as well as—or maybe even better than—common medications for diabetes like metformin and Actos," he said. "And it does this without *any* side effects."

A natural compound that works just as well as metformin, the most-prescribed drug for diabetes? Needless to say, I was intrigued.

Tell me *everything* you know about berberine, I said.

And Dr. Stengler proceeded to do just that.

A new use for an old herb

Berberine is one of the most active compounds in the herb *Coptis chinensis*, or Huang-lian, which is used in Traditional Chinese Medicine to treat people with diabetes, high blood pressure and heart disease, he explained. It's also found in the roots and stems of several other plants, including goldenseal and Oregon grape.

As Chinese medicine became less traditional and more conventional, Chinese doctors and scientists began studying berberine itself—the extract—rather than the whole herb.

They conducted cellular studies, showing berberine stimulated the production of AMPK (AMP-activated protein kinase). This enzyme improves the output of insulin (the hormone that ushers glucose out of the bloodstream and into cells)…helps muscles use glucose…burns fat… and also blocks the overproduction of fat. (Later in the chapter you'll read more about AMPK and berberine's mechanism of action .)

They conducted animal studies with diabetic rats, in which berberine lowered blood sugar, improved insulin sensitivity, and lowered LDL cholesterol—and did so better than metformin.

"Berberine displays an exciting anti-diabetic efficacy and may be of great value for the treatment of type 2 diabetes," enthused one team of laboratory scientists at the conclusion of their animal study in the *Chinese Medical Journal*. [1]

And then came the first studies on people, published in 2008.

Outperforming metformin

In one of those studies, 36 people newly diagnosed with type 2 diabetes took either metformin or berberine (500 milligrams, 3 times a day) for three months. The results were amazing. On average, those taking berberine had…

- Fasting glucose levels dropped from 191 to 124

- Post-meal glucose levels plummeted from 356 to 199

- A1C, a measure of long-term blood sugar levels, plunged from 9.5% to 7.5%

- Insulin resistance fell by 45%

Those taking berberine also had big drops in total cholesterol and triglycerides. [2]

How did those results match up with metformin?

"Compared with metformin, berberine exhibited an identical effect in the regulation of glucose," wrote the researchers in the journal *Metabolism*. "In the regulation of lipids [blood fats]… berberine activity is better than metformin."

Uncontrolled diabetes—controlled with berberine

The next study Dr. Stengler described was on 48 people with type 2 diabetes—people who were already being treated with insulin and with Chinese herbal formulas, but whose diabetes was poorly controlled.

The study participants were divided into two groups: one group took 500 mg, twice daily; the other took a placebo, i.e. a fake, lookalike pill.

After just two weeks, the folks on berberine had big decreases in the parameters of diabetes:

• Fasting blood sugar went from 172 to 135

• Post-meal blood sugar, from 266 to 189

• A1C, from 8.1 to 7.3

• Insulin dropped by 28%

• Insulin resistance, by 45%

"Berberine is a potent oral hypoglycemic [blood sugar-lowering] agent," wrote the researchers in *Metabolism*. "It is safe and the cost is very low." [3]

Beating Avandia

In 2010, doctors conducted a study comparing berberine to metformin and to Avandia. "Berberine's glucose-controlling performance was equal to Avandia and almost as good as metformin," Dr. Stengler told me.

"These were remarkable findings," he continued. "Here was a botanical that was holding up to scientific scrutiny—performing as well as, or even better than, drugs that diabetes patients had been taking for years.

"Berberine even *improved* liver enzymes, an indicator of liver health. Pharmaceuticals, on the other hand, have the potential to harm the liver."

Since those three studies were conducted there have been 15 other top-notch studies on berberine, involving more than 1,000 people with diabetes. In most of those studies, one group took berberine and another took either a diabetes drug or a placebo; in some studies, one group took berberine *and* a medication, and the other group just took a medication.

A team of Chinese doctors and scientists recently analyzed the results of all those studies.

Their conclusion:

"Berberine has beneficial effects on blood glucose control in the treatment of type 2 diabetic patients and exhibits efficacy comparable with that of conventional oral hypoglycaemics [glucose-lowering drugs for diabetes]." [4] And, they point out, berberine has "no serious adverse effects."

In other words, berberine is just as good as most diabetes drugs—and probably a lot safer!

How berberine gets the job done

Why is berberine so effective? "Berberine helps lower blood glucose in several ways," Dr. Stengler explained.

"It stimulates the activity of genes that manufacture and activate insulin receptors, which are critical for regulating blood sugar.

"It also activates *incretins*, gastrointestinal hormones that affect the amount of insulin released by the body after eating."

To delve even more deeply into the mechanism of action of this powerful natural compound, I interviewed Jianping Ye, PhD, one of the first Chinese scientists to study berberine in people with diabetes, and now a researcher at the Pennington Biomedical Research Center, at Louisiana State University System in Baton Rouge.

The key to berberine's effectiveness, he told me, is that it activates AMPK—a metabolic master switch. Once AMPK is turned on, the body can…

- Absorb more glucose (lowering blood sugar)

- Create more GLUT4, a "glucose transporter" that helps move glucose into muscle and fat cells   .

- Stimulate muscles to use more glucose

- Regulate the secretion of insulin by the beta cells of the pancreas

- Oxidize more fatty acids (burning up cholesterol and triglycerides)

- Limit the manufacture of cholesterol and triglycerides

- Limit the manufacture of fat cells

"Berberine is a very good natural medicine and dietary supplement, with almost no side effects," Dr. Ye said. "It improves glucose levels in the blood, reduces fat levels in the blood, and reduces body weight."

"Berberine is the unknown miracle drug from Traditional Chinese Medicine," agreed Angelo Druda, a practitioner of TCM in northern California. "Prior to the age of antibiotics, the Chinese used berberine-rich herbs to knock out strong systemic infections, reduce inflammation and balance blood sugar—and berberine can be used the same way today."

Powerful protection for your kidneys

Lowering blood sugar and blood fats aren't berberine's only talents. It can help protect your kidneys. And for people with diabetes, that means berberine can help keep you *alive*. Let me explain…

As I was finishing up this Special Report, a new study appeared from researchers at Washington State University in Seattle, showing that kidney disease kills far more people with diabetes than health experts thought.

The researchers analyzed 10 years of health data in more than 15,000 people. They found that 42% of those with diabetes had kidney disease, compared to 9% of people without diabetes. But here's what's even scarier:

The 10-year death rate for people with diabetes *and* kidney disease (31%) was nearly *three times higher* than for people with diabetes who didn't have kidney disease (11%). [6]

That's the very bad news. The very good news: berberine may protect the kidneys of people with diabetes.

There's no scientific proof for that protection in people. But there are about a dozen studies showing that berberine protects the kidneys of diabetic animals.

In one of those studies, Chinese researchers used a high-fat diet and a toxic drug to induce "remarkable renal [kidney] damage" in diabetic rats. Then they gave the rats berberine. Berberine completely restored kidney function and stopped damage to kidney tissues. [7]

"Berberine," wrote another team of Chinese researchers, "has widely been used for the treatment of diabetic nephropathy [kidney disease]." In their study, they treated diabetic rats with either metformin or berberine. Not only did berberine perform its usual feats of blood sugar control (lower glucose, lower insulin, lower A1C)—it also improved five biochemical parameters of kidney health. And when the scientists looked at the kidneys of the rats at the end of the study, those treated with berberine had kidney cells that were hardly damaged. "Berberine exerts an ameliorative effect on renal damage in diabetes," concluded the researchers in *Phytomedicine*. (In lay language: Berberine repairs kidneys damaged by diabetes.)

The doctors from Washington State University recommend "intensive risk factor modification" for people with diabetes and kidney disease, saying it's "likely to have the highest impact on overall mortality."

Well, if you have diabetes *and* kidney disease, one "modification" you should definitely consider is taking berberine.

How to use berberine

"I recommend berberine to my patients with newly diagnosed diabetes to reduce their blood sugar and prevent them from needing pharmaceutical drugs," Dr. Stengler told me. (He also recommends they participate in a comprehensive diet and exercise program.)

"Some patients are able to take berberine—and make dietary changes, like a low-GI, high-protein diet—and stop taking diabetes drugs altogether," he continued. "People with severe diabetes can use berberine *with* medication—and this combination treatment allows for fewer side effects and better blood sugar control."

The dosage he recommends: 500 mg, twice daily. You can find berberine online and in many retail stores that sell supplements. It's available in tablet or capsule form.

Dr. Stengler's final piece of advice (which applies to every supplement discussed in *Defeat High Blood Sugar – Naturally!*): "For patients with diabetes who want to use berberine, I recommend talking to your doctor about taking this supplement."

More doctors recommend berberine

Dr. Stengler isn't the only natural-minded MD to recommend berberine.

"Consider switching to berberine." "If you have type 2 diabetes and are being 'treated' with Januvia, Victoza or Byetta—all of which affect the incretin-driven blood sugar regulatory system—consider switching to berberine at 500 mg, three times daily," wrote Jonathan Wright, MD, in his *Nutrition and Healing* newsletter. "There's ample scientific evidence to support such a change!" (Like Dr. Stengler, he adds a caveat: "Make sure to work with a physician skilled and knowledgeable in natural medicine.")

"At the top of my list of recommendations if you have diabetes." Julian Whitaker, MD—author of *Reversing Diabetes* and medical director of the Whitaker Wellness Institute in Newport Beach, California—says berberine is the hottest new herbal supplement around.

"Berberine is poised to become one of our most powerful natural therapies for preventing and treating diabetes," he told me. "Plus, it can help with heart disease and with weight loss, and may even stave off dementia and other ravages of aging. Berberine is definitely at the top of my list of recommendations if you have diabetes."

Dr. Whitaker recommends 500 mg, 2 to 3 times daily. He adds this caution: "Although it is generally well-tolerated, it can cause constipation, which usually clears up over time, or with a reduction in dosage."

"The remedy that allows them to finally get off their medication." Fred Pescatore, MD—*New York Times* bestselling author of *The Hamptons Diet*—is super-enthusiastic about berberine.

"In many of my patients with diabetes, berberine is the natural remedy that allows them to finally get off their medication," he told me. "I would say the average drop in A1C is between 0.5 and 1%, which is comparable to metformin. It also helps control sugar cravings and helps people lose weight. I think it is a very unique agent in the treatment of diabetes."

Special berberine-containing formula: Dr. Pescatore recommends his patients use GlucoLogic, the berberine-containing supplement that he formulated. Three capsules daily provide 1,500 mg of berberine and also contain several other natural supplements featured in *Defeat High Blood Sugar – Naturally!*. A lot of his patients have been very pleased with the results…

Lower blood sugar and cholesterol. "I tried GlucoLogic because I'd read about berberine. I can't believe my blood sugar numbers have improved so much," said JT. "It also reduced my blood fats to within perfectly normal limits. It even increased my good HDL cholesterol."

Huge drop in A1C. "Since taking the berberine-containing supplement, my fasting blood sugar is at an average of 90 to 110, and my A1C went from 10.7% to 6.7%, said JG. "I have also lost 30 pounds in the last 5 months."

Ate sweets but blood sugar was still low. "This berberine-containing supplement is the best by far for controlling blood sugar," said LM. "It gave me low readings even when I intentionally ate sugar-sweetened things the night before."

43 years of trying—now something works. "I am in my 43rd year as a diabetic and I have tried many different products to help my diabetes," said GN. "I have found that GlucoLogic keeps my blood sugar much lower."

More anti-diabetes secrets in the next chapter...

• The new and startling scientific research linking *gut health* to diabetes—and all about *probiotics,* the digestive super-supplement proven to lower your blood sugar.

• The remarkable experiment in which probiotics lowered blood sugar from 191 to 117—reversing diabetes!

• The best type of probiotic for dealing with diabetes. (Not all of them work equally well.)

EXPERTS AND CONTRIBUTORS:

Angelo Druda is a certified practitioner of Traditional Chinese Medicine in northern California, and author of *The Tao of Rejuvenation: Fundamental Principles of Health, Longevity and Essential Well-Being.*
Website: www.traditionalbotanicalmedicine.com

Fred Pescatore, MD, is the *New York Times* bestselling author of *The Hamptons Diet* and several other books, and author of the Reality Health Check newsletter, which focuses on diabetes.
Website: www.drpescatore.com

Mark Stengler, ND, is a naturopathic physician, with a clinic in Encinitas, California and associate clinical professor at the National College of Naturopathic Medicine in Portland, Oregon. He is the author of more than a dozen books on health and healing, including *Prescription for Natural Cures, Prescription for Drug Alternatives* and *The Natural Physician's Healing Therapies.*
Website: www.markstengler.com

Julian Whitaker, MD, is the author of *Reversing Diabetes* and 13 other books on health and healing, and medical director of the Whitaker Wellness Institute in Newport Beach, California. He writes the *Health & Healing* newsletter for Healthy Directions.
Websites: www.drwhitaker.com, www.whitakerwellness.com

Jonathan Wright, MD, is the medical director of the Tahoma Clinic in Renton, Washington, and author of *Natural Medicine, Optimal Wellness* and 13 other books on natural health and healing. Website: www.tahomaclinic.com

Jianping Ye, PhD, was one of the first Chinese scientists to test berberine in humans, and is now a researcher at the Pennington Biomedical Research Center, at Louisiana State University in Baton Rouge.

RESOURCES:

The berberine-containing supplement, GlucoLogic:
To purchase GlucoLogic (or subscribe to Dr. Pescatore's newsletter), go to:
www.logicalhealthalternatives.com

REFERENCES:

1. Wei Z, et al. Anti-diabetic effects of cinnamaldehyde and berberine and their impacts on retinol-binding protein 4 expression in rats with type 2 diabetes mellitus. *Chinese Medical Journal*, 2008;121(21):2124-2128.

2. Yin, J, et al. Efficacy of berberine in patients with type 2 diabetes mellitus. *Metabolism*, vol 57, no. 5. pp. 712-717, 2008.

3. Zhang, Y, et al. Treatment of type 2 diabetes and dyslipidemia with the natural plant alkaloid berberine. *Journal of Clinical Endocrinology and Metabolism*, 93(70: 2559-65.

4. Dong, H, et al. Berberine in the Treatment of Type 2 Diabetes Mellitus: A Systematic Review and Meta-Analysis. *Evidence-Based Complementary and Alternative Medicine*, 2012;2012:591654.

5. Liu W, et al. Berberine reduces fibronectin and collagen accumulation in rat glomerular mesangial cells cultured under high glucose condition. *Molecular and Cellular Biochemistry*, 2009 May:325(1-2):99-105.

6. Afkarian, M, et al. Kidney Disease and Increased Mortality Risk in Type 2 Diabetes. *Journal of the American Society of Nephrology*, 2013, January 29. [Epub ahead of print]

7. Wang, FL, et al. Renoprotective effects of berberine and its possible molecular mechanisms in combination of high-fat diet and low-dose stretptozotocin-induced diabetic rats.

8. Wu D, et al. Ameliorative effect of berberine on renal damage in rats with diabetes induced by high-fat diet and streptozotocin. 2012 June 15;19(8-9):712-8.

Chapter 7

Probiotics

New finding:
friendly bacteria in your gut can help beat diabetes!

Don't look now, but bacteria have you surrounded. They're in the water you drink, in the food you eat—and they're inside your digestive tract, too.

<u>There are 10 times more bacteria in your gut than cells in your body</u>—about 100 trillion, a booming population scientists call the *microbiota*. (Bacteria are smaller than your body cells, so there's actually room for that many.)

What are all those bacteria up to?

Well, it depends on which one of the 1,000 strains of bacteria we're talking about. They're a complex mix of friendly and unfriendly microbes, with the good guys keeping the bad guys in check. But friendly gut bacteria—*probiotics*—do far more than keep the intestinal peace.

According to Liz Lipski, PhD, CCN—a certified clinical nutritionist in Atlanta, Georgia, and author of *Digestive Wellness*—those bacteria also…

- Balance intestinal pH (acid/alkaline balance)

- Reduce intestinal inflammation

- Digest milk sugar (lactose) and protein

- Manufacture B vitamins and vitamin K

- Break down bile acids

- Manufacture essential fatty acids and short-chain fatty acids

- Increase absorption of minerals

- Metabolize polyphenols, health-giving compounds in plants

- Break down and rebuild hormones

- Prevent food poisoning

- Break down and eliminate toxins

They also work to help prevent, control or heal a wide variety of conditions and diseases. These include:

- digestive problems like irritable bowel syndrome, constipation, diarrhea, flatulence, inflammatory bowel disease, lactose intolerance, kidney stones and liver disease,

- immune system problems like lupus, rheumatoid arthritis, allergies, asthma, eczema, bacterial and fungal infections, recurrent bladder infections, vaginal infections, and complications from antibiotic therapy

- heart problems like high cholesterol and high blood pressure.

Now, since this is a Special Report about blood sugar problems, you probably noticed that diabetes is *not* on Dr. Lipski's list. That's because scientific research linking diabetes to *dysbiosis*—the scientific name for runaway growth of bad bacteria in the intestinal tract—is very new: almost all the research on diabetes and dysbiosis has been published only in the last five years or so.

But I think you should know about (and act upon) the diabetes/dysbiosis connection—because restoring a healthy bacterial balance may be one of the most important (and easiest) ways to prevent, control or even reverse diabetes.

"There is tremendous potential for probiotics to impact diabetes," I was told by Steven Lamm, MD, an internist on the faculty of New York University School of Medicine and author of *No Guts, No Glory: Gut Solution—The Core of Your Total Wellness*. "When the body is inflamed, substances are released into the bloodstream that alter metabolism and affect the way we handle blood sugar," he continued. "It turns out that dysbiosis is a very important factor in systemic, chronic, low-grade inflammation. It's only a matter of time before health practitioners will start recommending probiotics for inflammation-fueled diseases like type 2 diabetes, obesity, heart disease and Alzheimer's."

For the readers of *Defeat High Blood Sugar – Naturally!*, that time is now—I strongly suggest you think about taking a probiotic to balance blood sugar. And I'm pretty sure you'll understand why I'm so enthusiastic about probiotics after you read the startling scientific story connecting gut bacteria and diabetes.

Bad gut bacteria: the secret cause of insulin resistance?

To understand the diabetes/dysbiosis link, you first need to understand *insulin resistance.*

Insulin is a *hormone*, a biochemical boss that tells organs and cells what to do. When insulin attaches itself to receptors on the surface of liver and muscle cells, it tells them to store *glucose* (blood sugar) as *glycogen,* a fuel the body uses for moment-to-moment energy needs. When insulin attaches to fat cells, it tells them to absorb blood sugar as *triglycerides,* a stored fuel.

But when those liver, muscle and fat cells are insulin resistant, sugar isn't absorbed—and blood sugar shoots up.

At first, the pancreas responds by pumping out more insulin—the boss raises his voice and the cells obey. Over time, however, the boss becomes burnt out, insulin levels drop, blood sugar stays high—and you're diagnosed with diabetes.

What causes insulin resistance?

Genes play a role, of course. So does a diet loaded with refined carbohydrates (soda, chips, cookies, white flour and the like), which wears out insulin receptors from overuse. So does a fatty diet, which clogs up receptors.

And so does dysbiosis.

The past couple of years have seen the publication of several scientific papers that review and summarize all the recent research on the diabetes/dysbiosis connection. They have titles like *Obesity, Diabetes and Gut Microbiota* (2010)...and *Gut microbiota and diabetes: from pathogenesis to therapeutic perspective* (2011)...and *Colonic flora, probiotics, obesity and diabetes* (2012)...and *Probiotics as potential biotherapeutics in the management of type 2 diabetes* (2013).

They detail several ways that unfriendly bacteria trigger insulin resistance (and also weight gain).

The bad bacteria...

• extract more calories from every meal (wearing out insulin receptors)

• store more calories as triglycerides (clogging receptors with fat)

• have a substance in their cell walls (LPS, or lipopolysaccharides) that sparks the immune system to produce systemic, low-grade, chronic inflammation, a known cause of insulin resistance. Scientists call this process *endotoxemia.*

- weaken the lining of the gut, causing *gut permeability* (leaky gut syndrome)—which allows inflammatory LPS to leak into the bloodstream.

On the other hand, the good bacteria…

- manufacture fatty acids (CLA, EPA and DHA) that reduce inflammation and fight insulin resistance.

- stimulate secretion of PYY (peptide YY), GLP-1 (glucagon-like peptide-1) and GLP-2. These three gut hormones help control appetite, balance blood sugar and insulin levels, and reduce chronic inflammation.

- strengthen the lining of the gut.

(Before we continue discussing diabetes/dysbiosis, I'd like to pause for a moment and emphasize that insulin resistance isn't only a problem in prediabetes and diabetes. All that extra insulin is toxic to your body, causing and complicating many health problems. "High levels of insulin resistance are the #1 cause of rapid and premature aging and all its resultant diseases, including heart disease, stroke, dementia and cancer," I was told by Mark Hyman, MD.)

Now, let's get back to diabetes/dysbiosis—and studies showing: 1) that dysbiosis is common in people with diabetes, and 2) that blood sugar levels normalize when bacterial balance is restored, either with probiotic supplements or a probiotic-rich food like yogurt.

Studies on probiotics and diabetes

"Accumulating evidence supports the new hypothesis that…type 2 diabetes develops because of low grade, systemic and chronic inflammation by disruption of the normal gut microbiota," wrote a team of researchers in *Diabetes/Metabolism Research and Reviews*. [1] Let's look at some of that evidence…

People with diabetes have different gut bacteria than people without diabetes. Researchers from Denmark studied 18 people with diabetes and 18 without the disease. Those with diabetes had a very different mix of friendly and unfriendly bacteria—and higher levels of particular strains of bacteria were a perfect match for higher levels of blood sugar. [2]

A probiotic supplement improves insulin sensitivity. In another experiment from Denmark, researchers studied 45 people with type 2 diabetes, prediabetes or no diabetes, giving them either the probiotic Lactobacillus acidophilus or a placebo. After one month, those taking the probiotic had better insulin sensitivity. [3]

Probiotics balance blood sugar in people who don't have diabetes. Finnish researchers started studying 256 pregnant women in the first trimester, dividing them into four groups; one group took a probiotic supplement during the second and third trimesters. (It contained the probiotics Lactobacillus rhamnosus GG and Bifidobacterium lactis BGb12.) Among the four groups, those who took the probiotic had the lowest insulin and glucose levels during pregnancy—and for a year afterwards, too!

"Improved blood glucose control can be achieved…with probiotics" even in a group of people with normal blood sugar levels, "and thus may provide potential novel means for the prophylactic and therapeutic management of glucose disorders," concluded the researchers in the *British Journal of Nutrition*. [5] (Translation: There's a new way to prevent and treat prediabetes and diabetes—probiotics!)

A combo of Lactobacillus acidophilus *and* Bifidobacterium lowers blood sugar—by 74 points! Researchers from Brazil studied 20 people with type 2 diabetes whose blood sugar wasn't controlled by drugs. They divided them into two groups: one group received a shake containing the probiotics Lactobacillus acidophilus and Bifidobacterium bifidum; one group received a placebo-shake.

After one month, those drinking the probiotic-rich shake had a huge drop in blood sugar—from 191 to 117. In other words, the probiotic shake *reversed* their type 2 diabetes—something that drugs couldn't do! They also had an average drop of 26% in total cholesterol, 41% in triglycerides, and a 35% increase in good HDL cholesterol. But those who drank the placebo-shake had no significant changes in either glucose levels or blood fats. [5]

Important: The shake also contained 2 grams of *prebiotics*, a type of fiber (fructooligosaccharides, or inulin) that nourish good bacteria. Several other studies show that a prebiotic supplement can lower blood sugar and increase PYY and GLP-1 hormones. [6]

The best probiotic supplements for diabetes

Not all probiotic supplements will produce the benefits you're looking for, I was told by Lynn McFarland, PhD, a research scientist in the Veterans Administration Puget Sound Health Care System in Seattle, and coauthor of *The Power of Probiotics*.

When choosing a probiotic supplement for healing, here's what to look for…

Match the strain to the disease. A particular strain of probiotics may not solve your particular health problem, Dr. McFarland said. Choose the strain that research shows can help the condition you're trying to prevent or treat.

With diabetes, that means taking a probiotic that contains *Lactobacillus acidophilus* and *Bifidobacterium bifidum.* For maximum effectiveness, you should also take a prebiotic containing oligofructose (inulin).

Buy from a reputable manufacturer. Dr. McFarland sent a variety of probiotic supplements to independent laboratories—and found that more than a third of the supplements didn't contain the type or amount of probiotics advertised on the label. "To get a quality product, buy from an established manufacturer that sells a wide variety of supplements," she said.

- The company Consumer Lab produced a similar result when they tested 25 probiotics—and 8 of them contained less than 1% of the number of probiotic bacteria listed on the label. Some of the brands that contained both lactobacillus and bifidobacteria (the diabetes-beating combo) and the actual amount of probiotics listed on the label included:

- 3 in 1 Natren Health Trinity

- Garden of Life Raw Probiotics

- Jarro-Dophilus EPS Enhanced Probiotic System

- Ultra Flora Balance, from Metagenics

- Nature's Way Primadophilus Optima

- Phillips Colon Health

- Probiotic Advantage from Healthy Directions.

In his book, *No Guts, No Glory: Gut Solution—The Core of Your Total Wellness,* Dr. Lamm recommends several manufacturers as reliable sources of probiotics. Among his recommendations, I prefer UltraFlora Balance, (formerly, UltraFlora Plus DF) from Metagenics, the company founded and led by Jeffrey Bland, PhD, who also founded the Institute for Functional Medicine—which focuses on treating the *underlying* cause of disease rather than symptoms. I trust Metagenics products for their purity and efficacy, and frequently suggest my clients consider taking them.

If you want to take a probiotic *and* a prebiotic, I suggest Prebiotic Inulin FOS, from NOW, a supplement company often endorsed by clinicians I interview.

Take a sufficient dose. For a probiotic to work, you need to take a lot of it—typically, about 10 billion organisms, Dr. McFarland said. That number appears on the label as 1/10(10)—shorthand for 1 times 10 to the 10th power.

Choose a refrigerated variety. "Probiotics come in two main types—those that need refrigeration and those that don't," said Dr. Lipski. "I generally prefer the refrigerated variety, because these delicate bacteria need refrigeration to ensure their life span and greatest potency."

Make sure you refrigerate them when you bring the supplement home from the store or get it through the mail, she advises. (Unrefrigerated supplements only lose a few percentage points of potency per week. But after several months of no refrigeration all the friendly bacteria are dead.)

Don't forget about diet

Probiotic supplements aren't the only strategy for supporting friendly bacteria.

Research shows that high-sugar, high-fat, low-fiber diets encourage the growth of bad bacteria—while good bacteria thrive on a diet rich in fruits and vegetables.

You can also increase your inner population of good bacteria—and your good health—by eating probiotic-rich fermented foods.

"There are a lot of great probiotic supplements, and I don't discourage my clients from taking them," I was told by Jennifer Adler, MS, CN, a certified nutritionist, natural foods chef, adjunct faculty at Bastyr University, and owner of Passionate Nutrition, a nutritional counseling service with six offices in the Seattle, Washington area. "But I also like my clients to get probiotics directly from fermented foods.

"That's because fermented foods have a large number of bacteria strains, and I think this diversity strengthens the digestive tract and overall health, compared to taking one or two strains in a probiotic supplement."

Adler advises her clients to eat fermented, probiotic-rich foods like:

Sauerkraut (unpasteurized, so the probiotics are active).

Kimchi, the Korean dish of fermented vegetables (which Adler likes to put on toast, with a fried egg, and a little mayonnaise and butter).

Kombucha, an effervescent ferment of sweetened tea. "It doesn't deliver as many probiotics as other fermented foods, but it fits better with many people's on-the-go lifestyle," she told me.

Kefir, a fermented milk drink with more probiotics than yogurt. "My clients typically preferred flavored to plain, which is often too tart for their taste," she said. "Because it's so rich in serotonin-boosting tryptophan, I recommend eating it right before bedtime if you have trouble with anxiety or insomnia." (In a study on diabetic rats, four days of eating kefir lowered glucose levels and decreased inflammation.) [7]

Another enthusiastic proponent of eating fermented foods for health is Donna Gates, bestselling author of *The Body Ecology Diet*.

"When you eat delicious, sour-tasting fermented foods, they dampen your desire for sweets—and controlling intake of sugary foods is crucial for controlling blood sugar problems," she told me.

Donna's company sells many high-quality fermented products, including: CocoBiotic (a fermented beverage from coconut); Potent Protein (a protein supplement, with a fermented blend of spirulina, beans and whole grains and flaxseed); and Kefir Starter (to turn milk into kefir). You can find ordering information for these products in the Resources section at the end of the chapter.

And then there's the fermented food that's easiest to find—yogurt. In a study on diabetes patients, eating ten ounces of probiotic-rich yogurt every day for six weeks lowered both fasting glucose and A1C. The yogurt-eaters also saw significant drops in total cholesterol and bad LDL cholesterol. [8]

When shopping for yogurt, look for a container with the words "live cultures" on the label, which means it probably contains a probiotic like Lactobacillus acidophilus. (Some popular national brands that contain live cultures include Activia and Yoplait.) Or look for the "Live and Active Cultures" seal, granted by the National Yogurt Association (www.aboutyogurt.com) to refrigerated yogurt that contains at least 100 million cultures per gram at the time of manufacture and frozen yogurt that contains at least 10 million cultures per gram at the time of manufacture.

Anti-diabetes secrets in the next chapter...

- Why one doctor calls green coffee bean "*the* blood sugar supplement par excellence."

- How to stop the formation of AGEs—toxic proteins that destroy the health of people with diabetes.

- Coffee is the perfect drink to *prevent* diabetes, says this expert. How many cups a day do you need? Find out in the next chapter.

EXPERTS AND CONTRIBUTORS:

Jennifer Adler, MS, CN, is a certified nutritionist, natural foods chef, adjunct faculty at Bastyr University, and owner of Passionate Nutrition, a nutritional counseling service with six offices in the Seattle, Washington area.
Website: www.passionatenutrition.com

Donna Gates is the bestselling author of *The Body Ecology Diet, The Baby Boomer Diet: Anti-Aging Wisdom for Every Generation,* and *Stevia: Cooking with Nature's Calorie-Free Sweetener.*
Website: www.bodyecology.com

Mark Hyman, MD, was co-medical director of Canyon Ranch for almost 10 years and is now the chairman of the Institute for Functional Medicine and founder and medical director of the UltraWellness Center. He is the *New York Times* bestselling author of *UltraMetabolism, The UltraMind Solution,* and the *UltraSimple Diet.*
Websites: www.drhyman.com, www.bloodsugarsolution.com
Facebook: facebook.com/drmarkhyman
Twitter: @markhymanmd

Steven Lamm, MD, is a practicing internist, faculty member at the New York University School of Medicine, director of Men's Health for NYU Medical Center, and author of *No Guts, No Glory: Gut Solution—The Core of Your Total Wellness* (Basic Health).
Website: www.drstevenlamm.com

Liz Lipski, PhD, CCN, is a clinical nutritionist, director of Doctoral Studies at Hawthorn University, and on the faculty of the Institute for Functional Medicine. She is the author of *Digestive Wellness: Strengthen the Immune System and Prevent Disease Through Healthy Digestion* (McGraw-Hill, 4th Edition).
Website: www.lizlipski.com

Lynn McFarland, PhD, is a research scientist in the Veterans Administration Puget Sound Health Care System in Seattle, and coauthor of *The Power of Probiotics* (Hayworth).

RESOURCES:

Probiotic supplement recommended by Steven Lamm, MD, author of *No Guts, No Glory*:
Metagenics: www.metagenics.com (800-692-9400) Product: UltraFlora Balance, (formerly, UltraFlora Plus DF)

Enter "UltraFlora Balance" into your search engine and you will find several websites that sell this product directly to consumers, including www.naturalhealthyconcepts.com (866-505-7501), www.drvitaminsolutions.com (888-432-5824), and www.vitacost.com (800-381-0759).

A website with high-quality fermented foods:
www.bodyecology.com

How to pick the best probiotic supplement:
I strongly recommend that if you're interested in taking nutritional supplements that *really* deliver what's on the label, you invest a few dollars a month in subscribing to the services of ConsumerLab.com, which identifies the best nutritional products through independent testing. Website: **www.consumerlab.com**

REFERENCES:

1. Panwar H, et al. Probiotics as potential biotherapeutics in the management of type 2 diabetes— prospects and perspectives. *Diabetes/Metabolism Research and Reviews*, 2013; 29: 103-112.

2. Larsen, N et al. Gut Microbiota in Human Adults with Type 2 Diabetes Differs from Non-Diabetic Adults. *PLoS One*, February 2010, Volume 5, Issue 2.

3. Andreasen AS, et al. Effects of Lactobacillus acidophilus NCFM on insulin sensitivity and the systemic inflammatory response in human subjects. *British Journal of Nutrition*, 2010 Dec;104(12);1831-8.

4. Laitinen K et al. Probiotics and dietary counseling contribute to glucose regulation during and after pregnancy: a randomized controlled trial. *British Journal of Nutrition*, 2009 Jun;101(11):1679-87.

5. Moroti, C, et al. Effect of the consumption of a new symbiotic shake on glycemia and cholesterol levels in elderly people with type 2 diabetes mellitus. *Lipids in Health and Disease*, 2012, 11:29.

6. Cani, PD, et al. Gut microbiota fermentation of prebiotics increases satietogenic and incretin gut peptide production with consequences for appetite sensation and glucose response after a meal. *American Journal of Clinical Nutrition*, 2009;90:1236-43.

7. Hadisaputro S, et al. The effects of oral plain kefir supplementation on proinflammatory cytokine properties of the hyperglycemia Wister rats induced by streptozotocin. *Acta Medica Indonesia*, 2012 Apr;44(2):100-4.

8. Ejtahed HS, et al. Effect of probiotic yogurt containing *Lactobacillus acidophilus* and *Bifidobacterium lactis* on lipid profile in individuals with type 2 diabetes mellitus. *Journal of Dairy Science*, 2011; 94(7):3288-3294.

Chapter 8

Green Coffee Bean Extract

You've heard about this "miracle cure" for weight loss. It might be miraculous for diabetes, too.

If you're a fan of health guru Dr. Oz, you may have seen the show in 2012 when he introduced his viewers to *green coffee bean extract*—calling it a "magic weight loss cure."

The extract is produced from raw, green, unroasted coffee beans—and Dr. Oz's enthusiasm for it was based on a scientific study reported at the American Chemical Society in March, 2012.

In the study, 16 overweight men and women…lost an average of 17 pounds…and 16% of their body fat…in 12 weeks…by doing nothing more than taking a green coffee bean supplement every day. [1] No dieting. No extra exercise. They just took the pills and shed the pounds.

Dr. Oz's report about the study—and hundreds of other reports in the media—unleashed a torrent of interest in green coffee beans.

But there's one thing Dr. Oz didn't say, the headlines didn't declare, and the countless folks who have taken green coffee bean supplements for weight loss probably don't know.

<u>Green coffee bean extract also may be an excellent supplement to prevent, control and reverse diabetes</u>—in fact, it works for weight loss *because* it's so effective at blood sugar control.

The anti-diabetic power of chlorogenic acid

"Slowing the release of blood sugar into the body is the key mechanism by which green coffee bean extract drives weight loss," I was told by Lindsey Duncan, ND, CN, a naturopathic doctor and certified nutritionist in Austin, Texas, who appeared with Dr. Oz on his first show about green coffee beans.

Dr. Lindsey (as he likes to be called) first discovered the power of green coffee beans when he was researching the antioxidants in the coffee cherry. ("Coffee is a fruit, and the so-called coffee 'bean' is the seed of the fruit," he explained.)

"I always thought coffee was damaging to health," he told me. "But while researching the coffee cherry, I started reading research showing that a component of green coffee bean—

chlorogenic acid—was more powerful than medication in lowering blood sugar in laboratory animals."

Chlorogenic acid (a collective name for a family of similar chemicals) is the active ingredient in green coffee bean extract.

Chlorogenic acid is a "triple threat" for extra pounds, says Dr. Lindsey: 1) it limits the absorption and utilization of sugar in the diet; 2) it blocks the storage of fat, and 3) it burns more fat.

All of which means chlorogenic acid makes green coffee beans remarkably anti-diabetic.

Here is just a small selection of the dozens of scientific studies demonstrating chlorogenic acid's power to deal with diabetes. The studies show the compound can…

Activate AMPK—the enzymatic master key to blood sugar control. Researchers found that chlorogenic acid activates AMPK—an enzyme that improves the output of insulin (the hormone that ushers glucose out of the bloodstream and into the cells)…helps muscles use glucose…burns fat…and also blocks the overproduction of fat. In the same study, the researchers found that injecting animals with chlorogenic acid dramatically lowered their blood sugar. [2]

Lower glucose and insulin. In an animal study, eight weeks of treatment with chlorogenic acid produced remarkable effects in animals fed a high-fat diet—lowering not only glucose and insulin, but also total cholesterol, LDL and triglycerides. The researchers also noted that chlorogenic acid activated PPARs—the same cellular target that several glucose-lowering drugs aim at. [3]

The human studies are just as impressive as these animal studies. French researchers gave a glucose tolerance test to 15 overweight men—who then took either 1,000 milligrams (mg) of chlorogenic acid or a placebo. Those taking chlorogenic acid had 29% less glucose and 38% less insulin—a sure sign their bodies were efficiently managing extra sugar. [4]

Stop the formation of advanced glycation end products (AGEs)—toxic proteins that destroy the health of people with diabetes. AGEs occur when extra glucose sticks to and alters proteins. Many experts think the buildup of AGEs is the main cause of the long-term complications of diabetes, like heart disease, kidney disease, blindness, nerve damage, and hard-to-heal leg and foot ulcers that can lead to amputation. In a study by Korean researchers, chlorogenic acid effectively inhibited the formation of AGEs—in fact, it performed far better than another "well-known AGE inhibitor." Chlorogenic acid, concluded the researchers, "could be beneficial in the prevention of AGEs progression in patients with diabetes." [5]

"It is the blood sugar supplement *par excellence*."

"My therapeutic epiphany with green coffee bean extract is that it's *not* a weight loss supplement—it's a blood sugar supplement," Dr. Lindsey told me. "It works by slowing the release of blood sugar into the body—and the side effect is weight loss.

"And it is *the* blood sugar supplement par excellence—nothing else even comes close for glucose control."

How much green coffee bean do you need to take to get your blood sugar under control?

√ Dr. Lindsey recommends 800 to 1200 milligrams (mg), 20 to 30 minutes before each meal. (Pills are typically 400 milligrams, so that would be two to three pills with each meal.)

√ However, he adds, drinking 10 ounces of water with every dosing is critical, because water activates the chlorogenic acid.

"I know green coffee bean can help diabetic and obese Americans," he said. "But it also works over time—you'll see more of an effect by the second month than you will by the second day. That's because your diabetes didn't develop in a day—it took a long time to do the damage to the pancreas and liver and other organs that resulted in diabetes, and it will take time to undo that damage. But over time green coffee bean is going to help your body function *really* well again."

Dr. Lindsey told me a few stories of diabetes patients where taking green coffee bean extract made all the difference.

"I've had hundreds of people tell me the supplement has made a tremendous difference in weight loss *and* blood sugar control," he said. "One woman with diabetes lost 28 pounds while on the supplement, and was able to reduce her dosage of insulin to almost nothing. Other people have been able to go off their insulin entirely, under the supervision of their doctors."

Beware of inferior products— and buy the best

After Dr. Lindsey appeared on the Dr. Oz show to talk about green coffee bean extract, a lot of fly-by-night companies started flying, putting up websites and sending spam to sell second-rate green coffee bean extract—some of which contained literally *no* chlorogenic acid!

"My team and I commissioned a third-party laboratory to test a selection of these brands," Dr. Lindsey told me. "One of them contained 0.04% chlorogenic acid—while the labeling on the bottle claimed the product contained 50%!

Many other brands also failed the assay—their labels advertising one thing and their product delivering quite another.

"It's a sad situation, because I have received so many emails and phone calls, asking 'Why aren't I losing weight on green coffee bean?' My first question is, 'What brand are you using?'

"You need to give yourself a truly fair chance with this incredible super-supplement by starting with a quality product that actually *contains* the key active ingredient, chlorogenic acid."

Dr. Lindsey recommends three products, two of which he formulated at his company, Genesis Today:

- Pure Green Coffee Bean, from Pure Health.

- Pure Green Coffee Extract, from Genesis Today.

- Green Coffee Bean, with Svetol, from Genesis Today.

(You can find purchasing information for these three products in the Resources section, at the end of the chapter.)

Dr. Lindsey's extract has these features…

Strength. The best extract contains at least 45% chlorogenic acid—and that's what you'll find in his two products.

Capsule form. Don't trust any product that's in tablet rather than capsule form, he told me: the heat used to process and create the tablet destroys the chlorogenic acid.

A unique blend of beans. The New Genesis formulation has a proprietary blend of Arabica and Robusta green coffee beans that delivers not only the highest dose of chlorogenic acids, but a big dose of other health-giving antioxidants.

Not too much caffeine. Some green coffee bean extracts are loaded with caffeine—and many folks find the extra caffeine makes them jittery or anxious or ruins their sleep. A daily dose of the New Genesis products deliver about 15 to 23 mg of caffeine.

(A typical 8-ounce cup of coffee delivers 100 mg.)

Purity. Dr. Lindsey's products are free of fillers, binders and artificial ingredients.

To Dr. Lindsey's list of recommendations, I would add green coffee bean extracts from two other brands:

- LifeExtension (Green Coffee Extract CoffeeGenic)

- Source Naturals (Green Coffee Extract).

That's because their products contain the same green coffee bean extract used in the weight loss study on green coffee beans, I was told by Joe Vinson, PhD, the lead author of the study and a professor of chemistry at Scranton University in Pennsylvania.

The brain-protecting power of chlorogenic acid

Recently, a team of researchers in the Department of Neurology at Mount Sinai School of Medicine in New York tested Svetol (another version of green coffee bean extract) in animals fed a high-fat diet. Not surprisingly, they found the supplement reversed insulin resistance caused by the diet. [7]

But it had a second and somewhat surprising effect: it also benefitted brain cells, powering up their mitochondria, the tiny structures that produce cellular energy.

"In our work at Mount Sinai, we have discovered that one of the first signs of the degeneration that leads to Alzheimer's—a change that precedes the onset of symptoms—is an impairment of energy metabolism in brain cells," I was told by Giulio M. Pasinetti, MD, the study's lead researcher, and professor of neurology, psychiatry and neuroscience in the Department of Neurology. "A supplement containing chlorogenic acid may be one way to prevent that impairment."

√ That's particularly important information if you have diabetes, which quadruples your risk of developing Alzheimer's disease.

Help for your heart

In the weight loss study that generated all the excitement about green coffee beans, the participants had a cardiovascular benefit that probably wasn't caused by shedding pounds: their average heart rate decreased by two beats per minute.

"I think that's the most surprising data from the study," Dr. Vinson told me. "And that drop in heart rate is a good thing. When you get older, your heart muscle gets older and your heart rate goes up—which creates the wear-and-tear on your arteries. And that's not just in people with heart problems—that's everybody.

"So green coffee beans might be an anti-aging supplement for the heart, too."

(Of course, Dr. Vinson is also keen on green coffee beans to prevent or control blood sugar problems. "It's definitely a glucose-lowering agent," he told me. "And it helps improve glucose levels not only in people with prediabetes and diabetes, but in normal people as well, making it preventive as well as therapeutic.")

Why not just drink coffee?

The beans used for coffee aren't raw, green coffee beans. They're brown beans that have been dry roasted. That roasting destroys a lot of the chlorogenic acid—there's simply not enough left to do the job of taming diabetes and obesity.

For example, in a study from researchers at the Harvard School of Public Health, people who drank five cups of coffee every day for eight weeks had *no change* in glucose levels or insulin sensitivity. [8]

However, there's enough chlorogenic acid in coffee to make it an ideal daily beverage for *preventing* diabetes.

In a review of 18 studies on coffee and diabetes, involving nearly 500,000 people, researchers found that every additional cup of coffee you drink reduces your risk of developing diabetes by 7%, compared to non-coffee drinkers. [9]

So, if you drink 1 cup of java your risk is down 7%...two cups, 14%...three cups down 21%, and so on.

And it doesn't matter if the coffee is caffeinated or decaffeinated—because it's the chlorogenic acid that's protective, not the caffeine.

"It could…be envisaged that we will advise our patients most at risk for diabetes to increase their consumption of…coffee in addition to increasing their levels of physical activity and weight loss," concluded the researchers in the *Archives of Internal Medicine*.

More anti-diabetes secrets in the next chapter...

• All about galectin-3, the newly discovered risk factor that can raise your risk of death *four-fold*—and modified citrus pectin (MCP), the super-supplement that can block it.

• The right dose of MCP for preventing blood sugar problems, for prediabetes, and for diabetes.

• The new, FDA-approved blood test that might save your life.

EXPERTS AND CONTRIBUTORS:

Lindsey Duncan, ND, CN, is a naturopathic doctor and certified nutritionist, and founder, CEO, Chairman of the Board and lead formulator of Genesis Today, a healthy super-food, beverage and snack company in Austin, Texas.

Websites: www.drlindsey.com, www.genesistoday.com

Giulio M. Pasinetti, MD, PhD, is a professor of neurology, psychiatry and neuroscience in the Department of Neurology at Mount Sinai School of Medicine in New York.

Joe Vinson, PhD, is a professor of chemistry at Scranton University, in Pennsylvania, and a renowned expert in polyphenols, health-giving compounds in plants (a class of compounds that includes chlorogenic acid).

RESOURCES:

To buy Pure Green Coffee Bean or Green Coffee Bean, with Svetol , from Genesis Today:
Go to the website:
www.genesistoday.com,
Or call: 1-800-916-6642
To find the product in a retail store, use the Genesis Today store locator, at:
http://superfoods.genesistoday.com/store-locator

To buy Naturally Pure Green Coffee Bean, from Pure Health:
Go to the website:
www.purehealth100.com
Or call: 1-888-323-9355
You can also find the product at Sam's Club and Wal-Mart stores

To buy Green Coffee Extract CoffeeGenic from Life Extension:
Go to the webpage:
http://www.lef.org/search/health-goal.weight-management/index.aspx

REFERENCES:

1. Vinson, JA, et al. Randomized, double-blind, placebo-controlled, linear dose, crossover study to evaluate the efficacy and safety of a green coffee bean extract in overweight subjects. *Diabetes, Metabolic Syndrome and Obesity: Targets and Therapy*, 2011:4 1-7.

2. Ong KW, et al. Chlorogenic acid stimulate glucose transport in skeletal muscle via AMPK activation: a contributor to the beneficial effects of coffee on diabetes. *PLoS One*, 2012;7(3):e32718.

3. Li Sy, et al. Modulating effects of chlorogenic acid on lipids and glucose metabolism and expression of hepatic peroxisome proliferator-activated receptor-alpha in golden hamsters fed on high fat diet. *Biomedical and Environmental Sciences*, 2009 Apr;22(2):122-9.

4. van Dijk, AE, et al. Acute effects of decaffeinated coffee and the major components chlorogenic acid and trigonelline on glucose tolerance. *Diabetes Care*, 2009 Jun;32(6):1023-5.

5. Kim J, et al. Chlorogenic acid inhibits the formation of advanced glycation end products and associated protein cross-linking. *Archives of Pharmacal Research*, 2011 Mar;34(3):495-500.

6. Thom E. A randomized, double-blind placebo-controlled trial of a new weight-reducing agent of natural origin. *Journal of International Medical Research*, 200 Sep-Oct;28(5):229-33.

7. Ho L, et al. Dietary supplementation with decaffeinated green coffee improves diet-induced insulin resistance and brain energy metabolism in mice.

8. Wedick NM, et al. Effects of caffeinated and decaffeinated coffee on biological risk factors for type 2 diabetes: a randomized controlled trial. *Nutrition Journal*, 2011, 10:93.

9. Huxley R, et al. Coffee, Decaffeinated Coffee and Tea Consumption in Relation to Incident Type 2 Diabetes Mellitus. *Archives of Internal Medicine*, 169 (No. 22), Dec 14/28, 2009.

Chapter 9

Modified Citrus Pectin

Galectin-3—a newly-discovered, toxic protein—is poisoning your pancreas. Modified citrus pectin is the only natural antidote.

Chances are, you've never heard of *galectin-3*, a protein discovered in the mid-90s.

But if you're concerned about your high blood sugar, it's time you learned about this compound, because it might be hurting you. Maybe even killing you…

Startling new scientific research: In a 10-year study, Dutch scientists analyzed health data from nearly 8,000 people. They found that those with the highest blood levels of galectin-3 also had higher blood pressure…were burdened with higher levels of artery-clogging blood fats… were fatter…and had weaker kidneys.

And more funerals.

Those with the highest levels of galectin-3 had a death rate of nearly 15% during the ten years of the study—compared to a death rate of 3 to 4% among those with the lowest levels. [1]

<u>In other words, if your galectin-3 levels are high, you're four to five times more likely to die</u>!

And if you're already ill with chronic heart failure (a damaged heart muscle that pumps an inadequate amount of blood), your levels of galectin-3 accurately predict whether or not you'll die within the next *year*…

In a study in *Circulation: Heart Failure*, a medical journal published by the American Heart Association, Dutch researchers looked at 1-year death rates in more than 1,600 people with heart failure. Thirty-seven percent of those with galectin-3 levels above 25.9 ng/mL (nanograms per milliliter) died within one year…20% of those with levels from 17.8 to 25.9 died within one year…and 13% of those with levels below 17.8 died within one year. [2]

The fact that galectin-3 levels are so predictive of hospitalization and death in chronic heart failure was behind the FDA's recent approval of galectin-3 blood tests for people with the disease. (The agency is also reviewing the galectin-3 test for people with diabetes. You'll see why in a minute.)

Okay, galectin-3 plays a crucial role in wellness and illness. But what *is* it, exactly?

Galectin-3, from normal to abnormal

As its name indicates, galectin-3 is a type of *lectin*: a protein that binds with carbohydrates, playing a variety of regulatory roles in the life and death of cells. When levels are normal, galectin-3 is a good guy, helping you stay healthy. But when levels rise (for reasons scientists don't yet understand), galectin-3 goes bad, turning into a kind of toxic glue.

It _inflames_ cells—the constant, low-grade inflammation that triggers and worsens chronic diseases, like diabetes, heart disease and Alzheimer's.

It fuels *fibrosis*, the brute transformation of flexible, juicy, living tissue into hard, dry, dead tissue—*scar* tissue—advancing heart disease, liver disease and many other health problems. (As you'll soon read, galectin-3 can cause both inflammation and fibrosis in the pancreas, crippling your ability to make glucose-regulating insulin.)

It makes cells more _sticky_, allowing cancer cells to form gangs and travel from the original tumor to terrorize other parts of the body, a process called *metastases*.

It's only in the last decade or so that scientists began to notice and start figuring out the importance of galectin-3 in disease. But now it's being studied in thousands of labs worldwide. Enter "galectin-3" into the search engine of the massive medical database of the National Institutes of Health (www.pubmed.com), and you'll get the results of nearly 2,000 scientific studies, linking the compound to heart disease…cancer…arthritis…liver disease…inflammatory bowel disease…asthma…chronic kidney disease…

And diabetes.

Let's take a look at some of those studies on diabetes, to understand the importance of galectin-3 in blood sugar problems.

And after we've taken a brief tour of that research, I'd like to introduce you to the only natural way to *stop* galectin-3 from harming you: the super-supplement, Modified Citrus Pectin.

High galectin-3, high risk for people with diabetes

There are lots of different ways that high levels of galectin-3 can cause or complicate diabetes.

Pancreatic cells die—killed by galectin-3. The beta cells of the pancreas manufacture insulin, the hormone that regulates blood sugar. The death of beta cells is a "hallmark" of diabetes, wrote a team of Serbian researchers studying the link between galectin-3 and beta cells in mice. They found that when galectin-3 was removed from the scene (either through breeding mice that didn't produce galectin-3, or through chemical treatment) beta cells stayed alive and functioned better after being challenged by inflammatory compounds.

Galectin-3 causes the death of beta cells in the presence of the chronic inflammation of diabetes, wrote the researchers in the *Journal of Cell Physiology*—concluding that the compound plays an "important role" in the development of diabetes. [3]

14% higher levels of galectin-3 in diabetes. Researchers in Germany studied 83 people— 23 were not overweight; 30 were overweight; and 30 had type 2 diabetes. They found galectin-3 was 14% higher in the people with diabetes, and 11% higher in the people who were overweight. [4]

In earlier studies, the same team of researchers found that galectin-3 was more active in the cells of diabetes patients…and that mice with lower levels of galectin-3 had less inflammation, smaller and fewer plaques in their arteries, and less susceptibility to diabetes.

Arteries are inflamed in diabetes—and galectin-3 plays a role. Mice receiving a high-fat, diabetes-causing diet quickly developed high blood sugar, inflamed arteries—and high levels of galectin-3, reported scientists at the University of Hawaii School of Medicine in Honolulu. "Elevated levels of galectin-3 support a role for this molecule in…diabetes, and its potential as a direct biomarker for the inflammatory state in diabetes," they concluded. [5]

Increased risk of eye problems in diabetes—because of galectin-3. Damage to tiny blood vessels in the retina at the back of the eye is called *diabetic retinopathy*—and it's the main cause of the vision problems that afflict nearly half of people with diabetes. In an animal study conducted by Irish researchers, blocking galectin-3 stopped those vessels from leaking. [6] In another study, diabetic mice bred to have no galectin-3 had far less diabetic retinopathy—their "inner blood-retinal barrier" was intact, wrote the researchers. [7]

Increased risk of kidney disease in diabetes—caused in part by galectin-3. Diabetic nephropathy—kidney disease—is one of the leading causes of disability and death in diabetes. Japanese researchers found more galectin-3 in the kidneys of people with diabetic nephropathy than in people with other types of kidney disease—and the higher the levels of galectin-3, the weaker and more diseased the kidneys. "Galectin-3 may play an important role in the progression of diabetic nephropathy," wrote the researchers. [8]

All of this evidence proves a very important point: at high levels, galectin-3 is very bad for blood sugar control and diabetes.

Now let's get to the good news I promised you: there's a natural antidote to galectin-3, a supplement that can lower levels of the protein and block its action...

Modified Citrus Pectin, or MCP.

MCP, the natural antidote for galectin-3

Pectin is a fiber found in the peels of apples, pears, plums, and in citrus fruits like oranges, lemons and grapefruits. (When an apple gets mushy, it's the pectin breaking down.)

In cooking, pectin is used to thicken jellies and jams. In industry, pharmaceutical manufacturers use it to aid the delivery of drugs to different parts of the body. In natural healing—because it can bind with compounds in the digestive tract and usher them out of the body—it's used to lower cholesterol. And because it's a *soluble fiber*—soaking up water in the intestines like a sponge—you can take a pectin supplement with a meal, feel fuller, eat less—and lose weight.

But that's pectin the way Mother Nature made it —big molecules, doing some heavy lifting in the digestive tract.

In the 1990s, scientists *modified* citrus pectin, creating a smaller molecule that could exit the GI tract and enter the rest of the body. Remarkably, a few cellular and animal studies showed that modified citrus pectin could battle *cancer*.

Fast forward to 2012.

A unique, patented formulation of modified citrus pectin with super-small molecules—PectaSol-C—has been shown to...

- help reduce the metastatic power of breast and prostate cancer cells

- spark the immune system to fight leukemia

- reduce a key biomarker of disease severity in men with recurrent prostate cancer

- reduce the growth and spread of breast and colon tumors in mice

- limit tumor growth and improve quality of life in patients with advanced stage cancer

- rid the body of toxic metals like lead, arsenic, mercury and cadmium, all of which might play a role in cancer

How does this form of modified citrus pectin work to battle cancer? Mainly by binding with and blocking the action of galectin-3, which fuels the growth and spread of the cancer—the same way galectin-3 fuels the development and worsening of diabetes.

An interview with Dr. Eliaz, the world's top expert in MCP

The scientist and physician who formulated PectaSol-C is Isaac Eliaz, MD, an integrative physician, licensed acupuncturist and homeopath, and medical director of the Amitabha Medical Clinic and Healing Center in Santa Rosa, California, which emphasizes the treatment of cancer.

"I would definitely recommend that a person with diabetes take MCP," Dr. Eliaz told me. "We know that diabetes advances because of inflammatory damage to the pancreas, and we know that one of the key players in this process is galectin-3.

"Plus, we know that galectin-3 plays a role in all of the degenerative damage in diabetes that occurs because of poor microcirculation and inflammation, including damage to the heart, kidneys, nerves and eyes.

"Because MCP can bind and inactivate galectin-3, it has great value in diabetes."

But Dr. Eliaz doesn't think people with diabetes (and cancer) should be the only beneficiaries of modified citrus pectin. "MCP addresses one of the main mechanisms of cellular damage and aging—high levels of galectin-3—and can help *everyone* prevent, control or reverse chronic disease," he told me.

The right dose with the best product

But, he continued, there are a lot of different modified citrus pectin products available—so it's crucially important to take the only type of MCP *proven* to lower galectin-3: PectaSol-C, from EcoNugenics. (You can find ordering information for PectaSol-C in the "Resource" section at the end of the chapter.)

As a preventive dose, Dr. Eliaz suggests taking five grams a day (in powder or capsule form), on an empty stomach.

(As an aside, that's the dose of PectaSol-C that I take every morning in 16 ounces of water, combining it with a citrus-flavored scoop of Energy Revitalization System, the daily vitamin-mineral powder formulated by Jacob Teitelbaum, MD, my coauthor of the book *Real Cause, Real Cure*. Why these two products? First, because they've been used in clinical studies that show they work. Second, because I've always been a big admirer and supporter of natural-minded physicians who see a critical need in their patients that isn't being met by any natural product on the market—and then use their experience and insight to create unique, powerful *effective* formulations that to meet the need. But back to the dosages…)

If you have prediabetes, he recommends 10 grams daily, in two doses of 5 grams, between meals.

If you have type 2 diabetes, he recommends 15 grams daily, in three, 5-gram doses, between meals.

Another way to determine dosage, he said, is to ask your doctor to order the BGM Galectin-3 Blood Test, which may be covered by your health insurance. LabCorp—a company with nationwide services—offers the test. Your doctor can learn more about galectin-3 testing at www.galectin-3.com. Once tested…

- If your level is 17.8 or above, take 15 grams.

- If your level is 14 to 17.7, take 10 grams.

- If your level is below 14, take 5 grams.

If the scientific studies on galectin-3 and modified citrus pectin are any indication, that daily dose may help you live a healthier, longer life.

Anti-diabetes secrets in the next chapter…

- Why a distressing *nine out of ten* people with diabetes are deficient in magnesium—and what to do about it.

- The exact amount of magnesium you need to lower your risk of diabetes—by a remarkable 75%.

- The best form of magnesium to take for blood sugar control.

EXPERTS AND CONTRIBUTORS:

Isaac Eliaz, MD, is an integrative physician, licensed acupuncturist and homeopath, and medical director of the Amitabha Medical Clinic and Healing Center in Santa Rosa, California. His company, EcoNugenics, is the patent holder for a uniquely effective formulation of modified citrus pectin, PectaSol-C.

Website: www.dreliaz.org

To order PectaSol-C, the form of modified citrus pectin science-proven to lower galectin-3:
Website: www.econugenics.com
Phone: (800) 308-5518
It is also available at amazon.com

REFERENCES:

1. de Boer RA, et al. The fibrosis marker galectin-3 and outcome in the general population. *Journal of Internal Medicine*, 2012 Jul;272(1):55-64.

2. van der Velde AR, et al. Prognostic Value of Changes in Galectin-3 Levels Over Time in Patients with Heart Failure: Data from CORONA and COACH. *Circulation: Heart Failure*, 2013 Feb 8. [Epub ahead of print]

3. Saksida T, et al. Galectin-3 deficiency protects pancreatic islet cells from cytokine-triggered apoptosis in vitro. *Journal of Cell Physiology*, 2012 Dec 31. [Epub ahead of print]

4. Weigert J, et al. Serum galectin-3 is elevated in obesity and negatively correlates with glycosylated hemoglobin in type 2 diabetes. *Journal of Clinical Endocrinology & Metabolism*, 2010 Mar;95(3):1404-11.

5. Darrow Al, et al. Transcriptional analysis of the endothelial response to diabetes reveals a role for galectin-3. *Physiological Genomics*, 2011 Oct 20;43(20):1144-52.

6. Stitt AW, et al. Impaired retinal angiogenesis in diabetes: role of advanced glycation end products and galectin-3. *Diabetes*, 2005 Mar;54(3):785-94.

7. Canning P, et al. Inhibition of advanced glycation and absence of galectin-3 prevent blood-retinal barrier dysfunction during short-term diabetes. *Experimental Diabetes Research*, 2007;2007:51837.

8. Kikuchi Y, et al. Galectin-3-positive cell infiltration in human diabetic nephropathy. *Nephrology Dialysis Transplantation*, 2004 Mar;19(3):602-7.

PART III

Nutritional Diabetes Cures

*Vitamins, minerals and other nutrients
for drug-free glucose control*

Chapter 10

Magnesium

Want to prevent blood sugar problems?
Take magnesium.

Let's cut to the chase: **Magnesium is *the* most important mineral for preventing prediabetes and diabetes**. And it's not bad for controlling less advanced blood sugar problems, either. Here's why…

The compound ATP is the fundamental energy source that powers every cell. But ATP is only half the story. It doesn't provide any power until it binds with magnesium to produce the molecule *magnesium-ATP*—the molecular motor for hundreds of enzymes, the sparkplugs of biological activities.

Now here's the kicker: many of those magnesium-dependent enzymes regulate *insulin*, the hormone that guides blood sugar out of the bloodstream and into cells.

When you have too little magnesium in your system (and research shows that most of us don't get anywhere near the amount we need), you're also likely to have…

- **low levels of insulin**—your pancreas can't produce the insulin your body needs; and/or…

- **insulin resistance**—your cells have a hard time making use of any insulin that's around, all of which leads to…

- **higher blood sugar levels**.

Magnesium is so important in balancing blood sugar, that one researcher—the late Ibert C. Wells, PhD, of Creighton University School of Medicine—theorized that <u>magnesium deficiency is the direct cause of one out of every three cases of diabetes</u>, and that simply by increasing your intake of magnesium, you could prevent or reverse the disease. [1]

Study after study says he's right—and that he might have even underestimated the diabetes-causing impact of inadequate magnesium.

Low magnesium = high blood sugar

Higher magnesium means lower glucose—in people who don't have diabetes. In a 2013 analysis of 15 studies involving more than 52,000 people who didn't have diabetes, researchers from Tufts University discovered an exact correlation between magnesium and blood sugar levels: the higher the magnesium, the lower the blood glucose. [2]

90% higher risk of metabolic syndrome (a precursor of diabetes)—with low magnesium. Metabolic syndrome is a constellation of health problems (including high blood sugar) that are often found together and that raise your risk for diabetes and heart disease. In a study of 441 people, those with low magnesium levels were 90% more likely to develop metabolic syndrome. [3] And in a study of 600 people, those with low magnesium were *six times* more likely to also have metabolic syndrome. [4]

49% higher risk of prediabetes—with low magnesium. In a 10-year study of more than 800 people, those with the lowest magnesium levels at the beginning of the study were 49% more likely to develop prediabetes (and more than twice as likely to develop diabetes). [5]

78% higher risk of diabetes—with low magnesium. In an analysis of 13 studies involving more than 536,000 people, researchers found that those with the lowest dietary intake of magnesium had a 78% higher risk of developing diabetes. [6]

77% of diabetes patients are magnesium deficient. When researchers analyzed magnesium levels in 51 people with type 2 diabetes, they found 77% were deficient in the mineral—and the lower their magnesium, the higher their blood sugar. "Magnesium," concluded the researchers, plays "an important role in blood glucose control." [7]

Complications multiply with low magnesium. Researchers at the School of Medicine at UCLA reviewed 80 studies on magnesium and diabetes, and concluded that a low level of magnesium is linked to *all* the typical complications of diabetes—heart disease and stroke; diabetic retinopathy (vision problems and blindness); diabetic nephropathy (kidney disease); diabetic neuropathy (nerve pain); and foot ulcers (which lead to amputation). "It is prudent to monitor magnesium routinely" in diabetes patients and treat low magnesium "whenever possible," concluded the researchers. [8]

(If you have diabetes, I'd say it's a lot more prudent to supplement your diet with magnesium so you never develop a deficiency in the first place. But more about that in a moment.)

Three times higher death rate in diabetes—in people with low magnesium. Critically ill diabetes patients admitted to the Intensive Care Unit were three times more likely to die if they had low magnesium levels, reported doctors in the journal *Magnesium Research.* [9]

But the dismal link between low magnesium and high blood sugar is easy to break—just take a magnesium supplement every day.

✓ **Take 500 milligrams (mg) of magnesium—and decrease your risk of diabetes by 75%.** In an analysis of 7 studies involving more than 286,000 people, researchers found that every additional 100 mg of magnesium in the daily diet lowered the risk of diabetes by 15%. [10] In other words, if you take a supplement of 500 mg of magnesium—a level recommended by many of the experts you'll hear from in a moment—you lower your risk of developing diabetes by 75%!

20% lower blood sugar levels in diabetes patients—after four months of magnesium supplements. A1C is a test that provides an accurate picture of long-term blood sugar levels. In a study of 65 people with diabetes, those who took 450 mg of daily magnesium for four months had an A1C of 8%—compared to 10.1% among study participants not taking magnesium. [11]

Those two percentage points translate into a lot of protection: for every one percent reduction in A1C, your risk of a heart attack is reduced by 14%, and your risk of developing eye, nerve or kidney disease is reduced by 40%.

Supplementing with magnesium: It couldn't be simpler

The evidence is clear: if you have blood sugar problems of any kind, you probably don't have enough magnesium in your diet. For example, in a recent study of 210 diabetes patients, *nine out of ten* had an intake of magnesium below the recommended daily allowance (RDA) of 400 mg a day. [12]

And the rest of us aren't doing much better. Research shows that half of all Americans get less than the RDA of magnesium. Magnesium experts I talked to for this chapter said the real level of magnesium deficiency among Americans is probably 70% to 80%.

How do you get more magnesium?

Well, it's smart to eat a magnesium-rich diet, featuring foods like whole grains, beans, green leafy vegetables, nuts and seeds. (Foods uniquely rich in magnesium include almonds, peanuts, cashews, brazil nuts, wheat germ, brewer's yeast, sea vegetables like dulse and kelp, and buckwheat and millet.)

But let's be realistic. No matter how good our intentions, few of us sustain a whole foods diet, day after day, year in and year out. Given that reality—and given the fact that you want to do everything possible to prevent and control blood sugar problems—taking a daily magnesium supplement is commonsense.

And choosing and using a magnesium supplement is simple, says Mary Block, DO, medical director of The Block Center in Dallas-Fort Worth, Texas, which emphasizes non-drug approaches in the treatment of chronic diseases like diabetes.

"90% of people who find themselves in a doctor's office need more magnesium."

"Magnesium is my favorite mineral," she told me. "I speak about it so much at medical meetings that some of my colleagues have started calling me 'The Queen of Magnesium."

There are a lot of vitamins and minerals. What got her so interested in this one? I asked.

"My son was diagnosed with type 1 diabetes 33 years ago, and I've been studying diabetes intensively ever since," she said. "In my research I found a tremendous association between magnesium and diabetes, both in type 1 and type 2. I suspect we'd see a whole lot less diabetes if we got a whole lot more magnesium.

"Plus, all the serious consequences of diabetes—the heart disease, the neuropathy, the eye problems, the kidney failure, the skin ulcers and amputations—are linked to low magnesium, and could be controlled by taking more of the mineral.

"In my opinion, every single adult in the world should take a daily supplement of at least 500 milligrams of magnesium—which would go a long way in preventing diabetes and many other medical conditions." (She also advocates 250 mg of daily magnesium for children, with a lower level if the child develops loose stools, a possible side effect of taking more magnesium than the body needs.)

"Unfortunately," she continued, "the role of magnesium has been ignored by our public health officials, and the role of calcium in health has been emphasized—even though taking too much calcium blocks magnesium!

"Well, a lack of magnesium causes depression, anxiety, high blood pressure, high blood sugar, menstrual cramps, muscle aches and pains, constipation and many other health problems—all of which are profitable areas for the pharmaceutical companies, which have so much power in setting health policy. So I'm really not surprised the official emphasis is on calcium, and that magnesium has been ignored." (You'll read more about the calcium/magnesium connection later in the chapter.)

"The public is not being made aware of the importance of magnesium—yet 90 percent of those who find themselves in a doctor's office or at the hospital are in need of more magnesium!"

Choosing a magnesium supplement

Point well taken, Dr. Block: We all need 500 mg or more of daily magnesium.

But what *type* do we need? There's magnesium ascorbate, magnesium citrate, magnesium sulfate, magnesium oxide, magnesium chloride, magnesium glycinate, magnesium gluconate, magnesium orotate and magnesium malate. (To name a few.) Is one better than another?

"I like magnesium citrate, glycinate or gluconate, because some of the other forms are more likely to cause diarrhea," she told me.

Her favorite brand of magnesium: Allergy Research, which is widely available on the internet.

Another magnesium expert—Carolyn Dean, MD, ND, a medical and naturopathic doctor, medical director of the Nutritional Magnesium Foundation, and the author of *The Magnesium Miracle*—agrees with Dr. Block that all magnesium supplements are not created equal.

Magnesium oxide is not well-absorbed, she says.

Magnesium citrate in powdered form, mixed with water, is best for people who tend toward loose stools when they take magnesium.

The company Jigsaw Health makes a good sustained-release magnesium with dimagnesium malate that also helps avoid any bowel issues, she adds. (See the "Resources" section at the end of the chapter for ordering information.)

Now about those loose stools…

A possible side effect: loose stools

There are two cautions if you decide to supplement your diet with magnesium.

Magnesium can cause loose stools or even diarrhea. If you take a 500 mg supplement and develop bowel problems, cut your daily dosage to 400 mg and see if the problem stops. If it doesn't, cut the dosage to 300. Repeat this process until you arrive at the dosage that's right for you.

On the other hand, some health professionals suggest you go in the opposite direction to figure out how much magnesium your body needs: Start at 400 or 500 mg, and increase the dosage by 100 mg per day until you develop loose stools; then cut back to the level where your bowels are normal again. (This is called dosing to "bowel tolerance.")

The second caution: Don't take magnesium if you have kidney failure. (For example, if you're on dialysis.)

The misleading magnesium test

Your doctor may have measured magnesium levels as part of a blood test and told you that you had nothing to worry about—your blood level was normal. (Normal ranges vary according to labs, but a typical normal range is 1.7 to 2.2 mg/dl.)

But a blood test for magnesium (also called a serum magnesium test) is very misleading, Dr. Dean told me. "Only one percent of magnesium in the body is found in the blood—making the blood sample a highly inaccurate reflection of your overall magnesium status.

"This test gives everyone a false sense of security about their magnesium levels. I believe in treating the person, not the test. The real question is, Do you have the *signs* and *symptoms* of magnesium deficiency? And metabolic syndrome, prediabetes and type 2 diabetes are three definite signs of a deficiency."

There are only two accurate tests for magnesium levels, says Andrea Rosanoff, PhD, co-author of *The Magnesium Factor* and director of Research & Science Information Outreach at the Center for Magnesium Education & Research in Pahoa, Hawaii. They are: 1) the Magnesium Challenge Test, and 2) the Exa Test, from Intracellular Diagnostics.

But, she told me, the challenge test is very complicated. (Even reading about it will be a little trying.) The doctor injects magnesium…you collect all of your urine for the next 24 hours… the doctor analyzes the urine, calculating the percentage of injected magnesium that was excreted in the urine…if you excreted less than 20% it's likely you have a deficiency, because your body was trying to hang on to the magnesium.

The Exa Test collects cells from underneath the tongue to measure magnesium levels in the tissue rather than the blood. It's a relatively simple test to conduct. But it's likely you'll have to convince your doctor it's the magnesium test worth taking (the cells can only be collected by a medical professional in an office). And it's only available from one laboratory in the U.S. (See the "Resources" section at the end of the chapter for ordering information.)

In most cases, neither of these tests is necessary, says Dr. Rosanoff. "Magnesium deficiency is so widespread, and a magnesium supplement is so safe to take, that rather than conduct inaccurate or complicated tests, it's better to just *take* magnesium and see if your condition improves after a month or so. Did your blood sugar go down a little bit? Did your blood pressure go down a little bit? If so, you *need* magnesium.

"And even that 'test' isn't absolutely necessary," she added. "If you have a health problem of any kind, you probably need more magnesium!"

Like Dr. Block, Dr. Rosanoff thinks that 500 mg a day is generally a good dosage, though you may need less or more, depending on your diet, health history, and bowel response.

The calcium connection

As Dr. Block said, calcium is one of the most popular supplements around—and you often find it packaged with magnesium, in a 2-to-1, calcium-to-magnesium ratio. But a lot of recent research shows that we're overdoing it on calcium. In fact, we're literally *overdosing* on it, with deadly results.

In the most recent study, involving more than 500,000 people, men who took 1,000 mg of calcium daily had a 20% higher risk of developing heart disease. [13] In another study, postmenopausal women taking calcium supplements were 49% more likely to have a heart attack and 37% more likely to have a stroke than women not taking calcium. [14]

Well, there's a reason they call a clogged artery "calcified"—plaque *is* mostly calcium. Taking a big dose of the mineral evidently hastens atherosclerosis, or "hardening" of the arteries. But there's another way calcium supplements cause heart disease: they lower your levels of magnesium, which study after study links to a healthier heart.

"Magnesium and calcium are like a see-saw," Dr. Dean explained. "If you take a lot of calcium, the body uses magnesium to neutralize it.

She says the oft-heard health advice of maintaining a 2-to-1 ration of calcium-to-magnesium in your diet is nonsense, based on an old-time recommendation that has no scientific support.

"The real ratio for optimal health is probably 2-to-1 magnesium-to-calcium," she told me. "Everybody needs more magnesium. Few people need more calcium."

The healthiest strategy, say many health professionals: Don't take more than 100 mg of calcium in a supplement. Get your calcium from foods. (If you're looking for non-dairy foods rich in calcium, try sardines, salmon, soy foods, dark green leafy vegetables, broccoli, sesame seeds, almonds, sunflower seeds, oatmeal, white beans, or dried figs. And take a magnesium supplement.

More benefits from magnesium

In her book *The Magnesium Miracle*, Dr. Dean says that, along with blood sugar problems, magnesium can help prevent or treat: anxiety…depression…high blood pressure…high cholesterol…heart attack…stroke…excess weight…premenstrual syndrome (PMS)…menstrual cramps…polycystic ovarian syndrome (POS)…infertility…osteoporosis…kidney stones… chronic fatigue syndrome and fibromyalgia…and asthma.

"Many of the miraculous magnesium stories that I hear involve heart symptoms, severe cramping, PMS, anxiety, and depression," she writes. "Most people with chronic fatigue syndrome and fibromyalgia improve about 50 percent when they begin to use magnesium. People who take magnesium for muscle spasms have said that their mild depression and irritability disappear as a wonderful side benefit. Invariably, people who take magnesium for one symptom find that it improves many others."

A quick trip around the web shows that folks with diabetes who take magnesium would agree with Dr. Dean…

Fewer leg cramps. "I have diabetes and terrible leg cramps," read a post at www. diabeticconnect.com. "The doc had me take a supplement with magnesium and that cut down on the cramps greatly!"

No more migraines. "I started taking magnesium because I was having migraines," says a post at www.diabetesforum.com. "I haven't had another migraine since—and that was about 4 years ago."

Weight loss. "I started taking a magnesium supplement a few days ago and I've lost 5 pounds already," says a post at www.marksdailyapple.com, by a woman with type 1 diabetes. "Couldn't believe it when I stepped on the scales this morning. I actually feel tons better too."

Helping high blood pressure. "I upped my magnesium a few weeks ago—and I really hope that my improved blood sugar and blood pressure are related to increasing my intake!" says another post at www.diabetesforums.com. (A different site than diabetesforum.com, above.)

Better sleep. "I am a person with diabetes who also has fibromyalgia and doesn't sleep well," says a post at www.healthboards.com. "I met someone in a pharmacy with similar health problems, and she told me to take magnesium to help me sleep—and it has worked since the day I started it."

And, of course, there's plenty of conversation about magnesium and diabetes…

Reversing prediabetes. "I believe magnesium deficiency was the main cause of my prediabetes—and I have been able to manage my blood glucose with the use of magnesium," says a post at www.lowcarber.org

. "I use a liquid ' ionic' form of magnesium from Eidon, and I love it—it has no diarrhea effect, and the amount that I take is considerably lower than most forms of magnesium." (This brand is widely available on the internet, or at www.eidon.com.)

Another post at lowcarber.org is equally enthusiastic: "I have been diagnosed as prediabetic and began taking magnesium. I kid you not, <u>my blood glucose is now within normal levels</u>."

Anti-diabetes secrets in the next chapter...

- The best dose of chromium if you have prediabetes or diabetes—as determined by the world's leading chromium researcher.

- Four, little-known causes of chromium deficiency. (If you recognize yourself on this list, you probably need more chromium.)

- All about brewer's yeast, the chromium-rich super-food. (Amazing scientific finding: It can lower blood sugar from 198 to 103—in just three months!)

EXPERTS AND CONTRIBUTORS:

Mary Ann Block, DO, is the medical director of The Block Center in Dallas-Fort Worth, Texas, an international clinic for the treatment of chronic health problems in children and adults, and the author of several health books, including *No More ADHD*.
Website: www.blockcenter.com
Phone: 817-280-9933

Carolyn Dean, MD, ND, is a medical and naturopathic doctor, medical director of the Nutritional Magnesium Foundation, and the author of *The Magnesium Miracle* and 30 other health books. She offers one-on-one phone consultations.
Website: www.drcarolyndean.com

Andrea Rosanoff, PhD, is the co-author of *The Magnesium Factor* and director of Research and Science Information Outreach at the Center for Magnesium Education and Research in Pahoa, Hawaii.
Website: www.magnesiumeducation.com

RESOURCES:

For an accurate magnesium test, which measures tissue (rather than blood) magnesium levels:
Intracellular Diagnostics, Inc
Website: www.exatest.com

For a magnesium supplement specially formulated not to cause loose stools:
Jigsaw Health
Product: Magnesium w/SRT
Website: www.jigsawhealth.com
Phone: 866-601-5800

REFERENCES:

1. Wells, IC. Evidence that the etiology of the syndrome containing type 2 diabetes mellitus results from abnormal magnesium metabolism. *Canadian Journal of Physiology and Pharmacology*, 86: 16-24 (2008).

2. Hruby A, et al. Higher Magnesium Intake Is Associated with Lower Fasting Glucose and Insulin, with No Evidence of Interaction with Select Genetic Loci, in a Meta-Analysis of 15 CHARGE Consortium Studies. *Journal of Nutrition*, 2013 Mar;143(3):345-53.

3. Guerrero-Romero F, et al. Hypomagnesemia, oxidative stress, inflammation, and metabolic syndrome. *Diabetes/Metabolism Research and Reviews*, 2006 Nov-Dec;22(6):471-6.

4. Guerrero-Romero F, et al. Low serum magnesium levels and metabolic syndrome. *Acta Diabetologica*, 2002 Dec;39(4):209-13.

5. Guerrero-Romero F, et al. Hypomagnesaemia and risk for metabolic glucose disorders: a 10-year follow-up study. *European Journal of Clinical Investigation*, 2008 Jun;38(6):389-96.

6. Dong J, et al. Magnesium intake and Risk of Type 2 Diabetes. *Diabetes Care*, September 2011, Vol 34, No. 9, 2116-2112.

7. Sales CH, et al. Influence of magnesium status and magnesium intake on the blood glucose control in patients with type 2 diabetes. *Clinical Nutrition*, 2011 Jun;30(3):359-64.

8. Phuong-Chi T, et al. Hypomagnesemia in Patients with Type 2 Diabetes. *Clinical Journal of the American Society of Nephrology*, 2: 366-373. 2007.

9. Curiel-Garcia JA, et al. Hypomagnesemia and mortality in patients with type 2 diabetes. *Magnesium Research*, 2008; 21 (3): 163-6.

10. Larsson SC, et al. Magnesium intake and risk of type 2 diabetes: a meta-analysis. *Journal of Internal Medicine*, 2007;262:208-214.

11. Rodriguez-Moran M, et al. Oral Magnesium Supplementation Improves Insulin Sensitivity and Metabolic Control in Type 2 Diabetic Subjects. *Diabetes Care*, Volume 26, Number 4, April 2003.

12. Huang JH, et al. Correlation of magnesium intake with metabolic parameters, depression and physical activity in elderly type 2 diabetes patients: a cross-sectional study. *Nutrition Journal*, 2012 Jun 13;11:41.

13. Xiao Q, et al. Dietary and Supplemental Calcium Intake and Cardiovascular Disease Mortality: The National Institutes of Health-AARP Diet and Health Study. *JAMA Internal Medicine*, 2013 Feb 4:1-8.

14. Boland, MJ, et al. Vascular events in healthy older women receiving calcium supplementation

Chapter 11

Chromium

Giving insulin a helping hand

The discovery that chromium is an essential nutrient—a nutrient that human beings can't live without—was a matter of life and death. Literally.

The year was 1977, and for the past three years a woman with a chronic digestive disorder had been receiving total parenteral nutrition (TPN), an intravenous solution that was (supposedly) meeting all of her nutritional needs. But—suddenly and unexpectedly—her health took a turn for the worse.

She lost 5, 10, then 20 pounds, and kept losing. She also developed severe *peripheral neuropathy*—nerve damage in the feet and hands, with numbness, burning and pain. This condition is common in people with diabetes, so her doctors gave her a *glucose tolerance test*, which shows how the body is utilizing glucose (blood sugar).

Her results were abnormal, and she was given *insulin*, the hormone that regulates glucose. But there was hardly any improvement. She was given extra glucose. Again, almost no improvement.

Then her doctors recalled earlier research showing that chromium can improve glucose tolerance. And because her TPN solution contained *no* chromium (it wasn't considered an essential nutrient at the time), the doctors theorized that a chromium deficiency might be causing her problems. Tests showed her blood levels of chromium were abysmally low: 14 times below normal.

The doctors added chromium to her TPN.

She began gaining weight. After two weeks, her glucose tolerance was normal. After five months, her peripheral neuropathy was gone.

Within the next few years, chromium was added to *every* TPN solution used in every hospital and clinic across America—because doctors and scientists had realized that chromium is an essential nutrient, and that a deficiency can cause severe disruptions in the body's ability to metabolize blood sugar.

Turbocharging your insulin

Since the late 70s, when it was discovered that chromium is a must for health, hundreds of studies have been conducted on chromium and blood sugar problems—with 78 scientific papers on the subject authored or co-authored by Richard Anderson, PhD, a Lead Scientist at the Diet, Genomics, and Immunology Laboratory of the Beltsville Human Nutrition Research Center, a division of the United States Department of Agriculture.

Chromium is a so-called *trace mineral*, present in the diet (and the body) in miniscule amounts, he told me. But it does a very big job—it improves the function of insulin, the hormone that moves blood sugar out of the bloodstream and into cells.

"When you increase the amount of chromium in your diet, you boost the activity of insulin," Dr. Anderson said. How does chromium give insulin a helping hand?

Every cell in your body has *insulin receptors*—tiny areas on the surface of the cell that let insulin latch on and send an important message to the inside of the cell: It's time to absorb glucose! Chromium *activates* an enzyme (tyrosine kinase) that helps insulin attach to the receptors. Chromium *deactivates* an enzyme (tyrosine phosphatase) that blocks the function of insulin receptors. Chromium also increases the number of insulin receptors. In effect, chromium turbocharges insulin—decreasing *insulin resistance* and increasing *insulin sensitivity*—and blood sugar levels drop.

As I said a moment ago, there have been hundreds of studies on chromium and blood sugar. Two recent scientific papers summarized the best of them. They found that chromium can…

Lower blood sugar levels in type 2 diabetes. Researchers from Tufts-New England Medical Center reviewed 17 studies on chromium and blood sugar control in diabetes—and found an average drop of 14 points in fasting glucose. And there was an average 0.6% drop in A1C, a measurement of long-term blood sugar levels. Both findings show chromium can cause a "significant improvement" in diabetes, said the researchers. [1]

Handle *any* kind of diabetes. In an article published in *Diabetes Technology and Therapeutics*, two scientists reviewed 15 studies on chromium, involving 1,700 people with many different types of diabetes—type 2, type 1 (an autoimmune disease), gestational (from pregnancy), and steroid-induced (a side effect from prescription corticosteroids). Every study showed that chromium *worked*—improving the body's use of insulin and balancing blood levels of glucose.

Are you deficient in chromium?

After 35 years of chromium research, Dr. Anderson is still enthusiastic about its ability to help balance blood sugar. But he's also quick to point out that chromium doesn't work for everybody.

Chromium doesn't work to *prevent* prediabetes or diabetes—study after study shows it has virtually no preventive effect, he told me. (Many other nutritional supplements are powerful preventives, like magnesium and vitamin D.)

And for people with prediabetes or diabetes, chromium works to balance blood sugar only if you're deficient in the mineral.

But if you have prediabetes or diabetes…and you are deficient…then chromium might play a role in lowering your blood sugar levels and stopping the advance of the disease.

Are you deficient? Well, that's not an easy question to answer.

Chromium is found in food in such teensy amounts to start with…and processing and cooking play such havoc with the small amount of chromium in those foods, making it even harder to obtain enough chromium from what you eat …and it's so hard to accurately measure chromium levels in the body…that the government hasn't even been able to establish a "recommended daily allowance" (RDA) for chromium. Instead, they use a more general designation called "adequate intake"—saying that 20 to 35 mcg is enough for adults. Are you in that range? You might not be if you're…

A dieter. A study showed that the Atkins, South Beach and DASH diet weight loss plans are all low in chromium. In fact, the study found that chromium was "nonexistent" in some of those plans. [3]

A senior. Lots of studies show that a chromium deficiency is common among folks 60 and older. One study looked at 12 people who lived at home and ate a "well-balanced" diet—yet all their diets were low in chromium because they didn't feature enough chromium-rich foods.

Not eating much brewer's yeast, wheat germ, calf's liver or oysters. Those are among the foods richest in chromium—and they're not staples of a typical diet. Other, more ordinary foods—whole grains, bran cereal, romaine lettuce, broccoli, green beans, mushrooms, tomatoes, potatoes, orange juice, grape juice, beer, wine, ham, processed meats, and black pepper—are decent sources of chromium. But not when they're overcooked, which destroys or removes the chromium.

Eating a lot of sugar and other refined carbs, which drains your body of chromium.

Bottom line: If you have prediabetes or diabetes, you *probably* need more chromium, so adding supplemental chromium to your daily diet may be worthwhile. "Personally, I think if you have prediabetes or diabetes, chromium is worth a try," Dr. Anderson told me.

The right dose for glucose control

Based on his decades of scientific research, Dr. Anderson's general recommendation for chromium supplementation is:

For prediabetes: 400 micrograms (mcg) a day, in three doses, taken right before breakfast, lunch and dinner.

For diabetes: 600 to 1,000 mcg, taken in three doses, taken right before breakfast, lunch and dinner.

Three, smaller, divided doses are far better absorbed and therefore more effective than one big dose, Dr. Anderson said.

And it doesn't take long for chromium to kick in. "Many studies show a lowering in blood sugar as early as three weeks after starting supplementation," Dr. Anderson said.

Which type of chromium works best?

The *amount* of chromium to take is one issue. The other is the *type* of chromium to take—and there are a lot of them.

For example, you can find chromium picolinate…chromium histidinate…chromium polynicotinate…chromium dinicocysteinate…multiple forms of chromium in one supplement… and chromium in combination with other nutrients, like biotin.

Is one type of chromium really better than another, as some scientists (and marketers) claim?

Well, you can find studies that support the efficacy of just about any form of chromium, Dr. Anderson told me. The final choice will be based on your personal perspective on the scientific findings…your personal experience with the supplements…and the advice and guidance of a heath professional. Here is some of the standout research on various types of chromium…

 Chromium dinicocysteinate. There's a new form of chromium on the block: chromium dinicocysteinate, sold under the brand name Zychrome.

The head of research at the manufacturer, InterHealth, told me that scientists working with the company tested a dozen different types of chromium over several years, looking for the one with the greatest effectiveness in managing blood sugar—and research showed this was the best.

In a recent study, 74 diabetes patients were divided into three groups: 24 took chromium dinicocysteinate; 25 chromium picolinate; and 25 a placebo. After three months, there was no difference in fasting glucose or A1C levels between those taking the two forms of chromium. But those taking Zychrome had much lower levels of insulin and less inflammation and oxidation, three signs the disease was better controlled. [5]

"This supplement combines two beneficial compounds. The first is chromium and the second is L-cysteine, which is itself a precursor of glutathione and hydrogen sulfide, two powerful antioxidants," I was told by Sushil Jain, PhD, a professor at the Louisiana State University Health Sciences Center and School of Medicine. "Each of these compounds can potentially enhance the effects of the other."

You can find chromium dinicocysteinate in: Zychrome Chromium Di-Nicocysteinate, from Swanson Ultra; Zychrome 400 from Progressive Laboratories; and Zychrome, from Wonder Laboratories.

Chromium histidinate. Research by Dr. Anderson shows this form of chromium is better absorbed than chromium picolinate, boosting blood levels 43% higher. [6] Several studies of diabetic animals have looked at a combination of histidinate and picolinate and found reduced inflammation and greater protection from damage to the brain and kidneys than picolinate alone.

You can find chromium histidinate and chromium picolinate in Chromax Plus Ultra Strength from Iceland Health, a division of Nutrition 21.

Chromium and biotin. Chromium and biotin (a B-vitamin) is a combination marketed under a wide variety of brands. Biotin is known to strengthen the insulin-producing cells of the pancreas and boost insulin production; the theory is that taking the two ingredients together is more effective than taking either one alone.

In a study of the combination, 447 people with poorly controlled diabetes took either Diachrome, from Nutrition 21 (600 mcg of chromium picolinate and 2 mg of biotin) or a placebo. After three months, those who started the study with an A1C higher than 10% had a drop of 1.76%—a bigger drop than that achieved by many drugs. (And that drop was among people who were *already* taking medications to control their diabetes.) "This study shows that adding Diachrome to antidiabetic medications can help patients reach their blood sugar goal simply, effectively and safely," I was told by Cesar Albarracin, MD, a Texas-based physician who led the study.

Chromium and cinnamon. Another frequently sold combo is chromium and cinnamon, an anti-diabetes duo endorsed by Dr. Anderson, who is arguably the world's top scientific expert in the glucose-regulating powers of chromium *and* of cinnamon. (He thinks cinnamon is more powerful. More on this to come in Chapter 16.)

In a scientific paper published in the *Proceedings of the Nutrition Society*, Dr. Anderson pointed out that both compounds improve insulin sensitivity (the ability of cells to respond to insulin), and have "similar effects on insulin signaling and glucose control." [7]

The most studied cinnamon supplement is Cinsulin, a water extract of the spice; it is combined with chromium picolinate and vitamin D3 in the product Advanced Strength Cinsulin, from TruNature.

Chromium is safe

Whatever form of supplemental chromium you choose, you can confidently rely on its safety, in spite of widely disseminated assertions that chromium picolinate may cause DNA damage, possibly leading to cancer.

"There is one study which showed some chromosomal damage from chromium picolinate in laboratory animals, but it was based on an extreme manipulation of scientific conditions and has no bearing whatsoever in the real world of human nutrition," Dr. Anderson assured me. "Chromium is safer than *water*. If you take 100 times more water than the body needs, you can die. If you take 100 times more chromium than is physiologically necessary, you can get healthier."

Brewer's yeast: a chromium-rich super-food

Safety issues aside, you may want to pass on the supplement and use a chromium-rich food instead: brewer's yeast. One tablespoon delivers 60 mcg of chromium, compared to 11 mcg from ½ cup of broccoli and 8 mcg from 1 cup of grape juice.

In a recent study with remarkable results, 40 people with newly diagnosed type 2 diabetes received either brewer's yeast or a placebo. After three months, those taking brewer's yeast saw a huge drop in the average blood sugar level from 198 to 103…and a huge drop of A1C from 9.5% to 6.9%. They also saw reductions in bad LDL cholesterol and triglycerides. [8]

Those results don't surprise Jacob Teitelbaum, MD, a natural-minded physician based in Hawaii, and co-author with me of the book *Real Cause, Real Cure*. He told me about a study conducted by a colleague which showed that adding two heaping tablespoons a day of brewer's yeast to the diet lowered blood sugar by 40%—the type of amazing decrease seen in the study I just reported, where glucose levels fell by 48%. Dr. Teitelbaum is convinced that there are many more nutritional factors in brewer's yeast than chromium that account for its power to control blood sugar.

Chromium is good for the brain, too

Brain cells are loaded with insulin receptors—and insulin resistance has been linked to Alzheimer's disease, I was told by Robert Krikorian, PhD, an associate professor of Clinical Psychiatry and Director of the Division of Psychology at the University of Cincinnati College of Medicine. "Insulin resistance causes high insulin levels in the brain, which drives neurodegeneration—which means that improving insulin resistance might help control mental decline."

That's why Dr. Krikorian conducted a study to see if insulin-enhancing chromium might improve the mental abilities and brain health of 26 older people with mild cognitive impairment, the stage of memory loss and mental decline that precedes Alzheimer's. [9]

Brain scans showed that three months of daily supplementation with 1000 mg of chromium picolinate increased activity in parts of the brain involved with memory. Written tests showed improvement in several mental functions that play a role in memory and learning.

"I recommend that older people with mental decline take at least 400 mcg of chromium daily, which is a very safe level of supplementation" he told me. He also advices them to reduce processed carbs and increase the intake of fruits and vegetables…take 1 gram of fish oil with an EPA/DHA ration of 2-to-1…take 100 mg of alpha lipoic acid before each meal…and take 2,000 IU of vitamin D daily.

Worldwide kudos for chromium

Chromium's ability to balance blood sugar has earned it many dotcom commendations:

Her three siblings have diabetes—but she doesn't. "I have taken 200 mcg of chromium along with biotin for several years," says a post at www.sparkpeople.com. "I'm 66 and three of my 4 siblings are diabetic and my blood sugar runs in the 90s—but I am not prediabetic. I have no scientific proof but I feel these supplements have helped keep my blood sugar even."

Chromium normalized blood sugar. "I had a friend who thought she was diabetic and the doctor ran all sorts of tests and found that she was chromium deficient," says a post at www.healthexpertadvice.org. "She was put on a chromium supplement—and her blood sugar is now down under normal levels."

Chromium/cinnamon combo is working for her. "I've been on meds for diabetes for 11 years—and I'm now in the process of cutting back on some meds with my endocrinologist observing," says a post on www.diabeticconnect.com. "I increased my exercise, cut back on carbs—and added a chromium and cinnamon supplement, and Aloe Vera juice to my regimen.

Those three additions are making a large difference, or so it appears—<u>my blood glucose is frequently in the 90s. That is better than my numbers were before I cut my meds!</u>"

More enthusiasm for chromium *and* cinnamon. "I have been using cinnamon for some time now and it has worked well in helping me control blood sugar," says a post at <u>www. peoplespharmacy.com</u>. "Recently, I started taking cinnamon *with* chromium—two capsules a day gives me 2,000 mg of cinnamon and 200 mcg of chromium, and this has made a big difference in my blood glucose levels. <u>I finally feel like I have found something that will naturally help me control my diabetes.</u>"

"Rages" from low blood sugar—controlled with chromium. "I am not taking chromium because of diabetes—I get 'rages' from low blood sugar that are difficult if not impossible to control, and have put strains on relationships," says a post at <u>www.bluelight.ru</u>. "<u>Taking chromium once a day has helped *dramatically*</u>."

Lowest blood sugar in 10 years. "In April I started both chromium and fish oil," says a post at <u>www.kickas.org</u>. "<u>Last month my blood sugar was down to 87—and it hasn't been that low in over 10 years</u>. I'm assuming it was either the fish oil or the chromium that did the trick."

Anti-diabetes secrets in the next chapter...

- How just a *small* boost in blood levels of vitamin D can *prevent* prediabetes from becoming diabetes.

- Why the world's top expert in vitamin D says the blood level of the nutrient recommended by the government's Institute of Medicine is a level that *causes* diabetes—and the blood level that's truly protective.

- The optimal dose of vitamin D. (There's a lot of differing opinions out there. I've made sense of them for you.)

EXPERTS AND CONTRIBUTORS:

Cesar Albarracin, MD, is a physician in Corpus Christi, Texas.

Richard Anderson, PhD, is a Lead Scientist in the Diet, Genomics, and Immunology Laboratory of the Beltsville Human Nutrition Research Center, a division of the United States Department of Agriculture.

Sushil Jain, PhD, is a professor of Molecular and Cellular Physiology and of Biochemistry and Molecular Biology at the Louisiana State University Health Sciences Center-School of Medicine, in Shreveport, Louisiana.

Robert Krikorian, PhD, is an associate professor of Clinical Psychiatry and Director of the Division of Psychology at the University of Cincinnati College of Medicine.

Jacob Teitelbaum, MD, is a board certified internist and Medical Director of the national Fibromyalgia and Fatigue Centers and Chronicity. He is author of the popular free iPhone application *Cures A-Z,* and author of the bestselling book *From Fatigued to Fantastic!,* as well as *Pain Free 1-2-3* (McGraw-Hill), *Three Steps to Happiness: Healing Through Joy* and *Beat Sugar Addiction NOW!.* His newest book is *Real Cause, Real Cure.*
Website: www.endfatigue.com

REFERENCES:

1. Balk EM, et al. Effect of Chromium Supplementation on Glucose Metabolism and Lipids. *Diabetes Care*, Volume 30, Number 8, August 2007, 2154-2163.

2. Broadhurst CL, et al. Clinical studies on chromium picolinate supplementation in diabetes mellitus—a review. *Diabetes Technology and Therapeutics*, 2006 Dec;8(6):677-87.

3. Calton JB. Prevalence of micronutrient deficiency in popular diet plans. *Journal of the International Society of Sports Nutrition*, 2010 Jun 10;7:24.

4. Basaki M, et al. Zinc, copper, iron, and chromium concentrations in young patients with type 2 diabetes mellitus. *Biological Trace Element Research*, 2012 Aug;148(2):161-4.

5. Sushil K, et al. Effect of chromium dinicocysteinate supplementation on circulating levels

of insulin, TNF-alpha, oxidative stress, and insulin resistance in type 2 diabetic subjects: randomized, double-blind, placebo-controlled study. *Molecular Nutrition & Food Research*, 2012 Aug;56(8):1333-41.

6. Anderson RA, et al. Stability and absorption of chromium and absorption of chromium histidinate complexes by humans. *Biological Trace Element Research*, 2004 Dec;101(3):211-8.

7. Anderson, RA. Chromium and polyphenols from cinnamon improve insulin sensitivity. *Proceedings of the Nutrition Society*, 2008 Feb;67(1):48-53.

8. Sharma S, et al. Beneficial effect of chromium supplementation on glucose, HbA1C and lipid variables in individuals with newly onset type 2 diabetes. *Journal of Trace Elements in Medicine and Biology*. 2011 Jul;25(3):149-53.

9. Krikorian R, et al. Improved cognitive-cerebral function in older adults with chromium supplementation. *Nutritional Neuroscience*, 2010 Jun;13(3):116-22.

Chapter 12

Vitamin D

The nutrient that stops diabetes in its tracks

I trust Paula Vetter, RN—a nurse practitioner, certified diabetes educator, certified herbalist, and wellness coach, with more than 30 years' experience in traditional and holistic medicine—to do the right thing for people with diabetes.

The *natural* thing…the *healing* thing…the thing that will *really* stop or reverse the disease.

So when I asked Paula for her recommendations for super-supplements for diabetes, I wasn't surprised that vitamin D—the "sunshine vitamin," formed when rays of sunlight hit the skin—was at the very top of her list. Because I'd been reading study after study showing the nutrient was very important in balancing blood sugar.

"Vitamin D is absolutely *crucial* in diabetes," she said. "It functions more like a hormone than a vitamin—and it does amazing things. It makes the cell wall more permeable to both insulin and glucose, lowering insulin resistance and high blood sugar. And it lowers inflammation, which is the root cause of diabetes and the factor that worsens it day by day and year after year."

Vetter isn't the only health professional who likes to praise the anti-diabetes power of vitamin D…

The twin epidemics: diabetes and vitamin D deficiency

The acknowledged #1 vitamin D expert in the world is Michael Holick, MD, PhD, professor of medicine at Boston University Medical Center, and author of *The Vitamin D Solution*. Like Vetter, Dr. Holick told me that vitamin D is crucial in preventing or controlling blood sugar problems. And he said the same to the international scientific community, in the article, "D-iabetes and D-eath D-efying vitamin D," published in *Nature Reviews/Endocrinology* in 2012. [1]

Here is his perspective on vitamin D and diabetes, which I've compiled from my many interviews with him, this recent paper, and his book…

"It's no coincidence that type 2 diabetes *and* vitamin D deficiency are epidemics—that

105 million Americans have prediabetes or diabetes; and that 70 percent of whites, 90 percent of Hispanics and 97 percent of blacks have insufficient blood levels of vitamin D. The two are inextricably linked." How? I asked.

"The insulin-producing beta calls of the pancreas have a vitamin D receptor," he explained. "And the production of insulin—the hormone that helps control blood sugar—is improved when beta-cells are exposed to vitamin D.

"In addition, scientific research links *low* blood levels of vitamin D to impaired insulin secretion, to insulin resistance, and to the metabolic syndrome. These scientific data strongly implicate vitamin D deficiency as a significant risk factor for type 2 diabetes—but the data has been ignored." (Keep in mind that metabolic syndrome and prediabetes are essentially the same thing.)

He points to several large studies that prove his point…

Lower levels of vitamin D, higher risk of metabolic syndrome. In a five-year study of more than 4,000 middle-aged people, those with low blood levels of vitamin D (23 ng/ml or lower) were up to 74% more likely to develop the metabolic syndrome than people with higher levels (34 or higher). [2]

More vitamin D—and prediabetes *doesn't* become diabetes. In a 10-year study of more than 2,000 people with prediabetes, those with the highest blood levels of vitamin D at the beginning of the study had a 62% lower risk of developing diabetes. [3]

"This translates," Dr. Holick said, "into a *remarkable* reduction in the incidence of type 2 diabetes among study participants with prediabetes—for women, a 21% lower risk per every 4 ng/ml increase in vitamin D blood levels; for men, a 27% lower risk per every 4 ng/ml increase."

Less vitamin D—and more heart disease in people with insulin resistance. In a study of 1,801 people with metabolic syndrome, those who had decent blood levels of vitamin D had 66% fewer deaths from heart attacks and strokes…76% fewer deaths from chronic heart failure…and 75% fewer deaths from any cause. [4]

(Why is this so important? Because as I've said throughout this Special Report, more than 80% of people with diabetes die from heart disease. So anything you can do to protect yourself from heart disease, you should do. And as you've just read, vitamin D is wonderfully protective.)

Teens are at risk, too. Dr. Holick points out that an estimated 50 million teenagers in the US are vitamin D-deficient (below 20 ng/mL) or vitamin D "insufficient" (20 to 29)—and that the deficiency is linked to a 2.5-fold increased risk of high blood sugar and 4.0-fold increased risk of the metabolic syndrome. [5]

"Improvement in vitamin D status should be a priority," Dr. Holick concludes.

Vitamin D: a healing force in diabetes

Dr. Holick's review on vitamin D and diabetes was published in July, 2012. I'd like to report just a few of the many studies on vitamin D and *healing* blood sugar problems that were published while I was writing this Special Report...

Less insulin resistance and lower blood sugar—with 50,000 IU a week of vitamin D. One hundred people with type 2 diabetes took 50,000 IU of vitamin D weekly for two months—and saw an average 9 point drop in fasting glucose...a 2.1 drop in insulin ...and an 0.68 drop in insulin resistance. "Vitamin D supplementation could reduce insulin resistance in type 2 diabetes," concluded the researchers. [6]

Healthier beta-cells—with 2,000 IU a day of vitamin D. In a study of 92 people with type 2 diabetes, a daily supplement of 2,000 IU of vitamin D improved the insulin-producing power of beta-cells in the pancreas—and also lowered artery-clogging LDL and cholesterol. [7]

Healing diabetic neuropathy—with vitamin D. A doctor at the University of Alabama Medical School had a patient with diabetic neuropathy (nerve pain) so severe he couldn't work. The patient also had a vitamin D deficiency—and when the doctor corrected it with vitamin D supplementation the patient's "symptoms improved dramatically." [8]

That finding wouldn't have surprised another team of doctors who found that their diabetes patients with peripheral neuropathy were three times more likely to have a vitamin D deficiency compared to diabetes patients without neuropathy. [9]

Healthier kidneys in diabetes patients—courtesy of vitamin D. Low vitamin D levels are common in diabetes patients with kidney problems, found Chinese researchers—but when they gave those patients daily vitamin D supplements, their kidney function improved. [10]

Leaner, healthier livers—with more vitamin D. If you have prediabetes or diabetes, it's pretty likely you've also got non-alcoholic fatty liver disease (NAFLD)—a buildup of fat in the liver that can cause inflammation and scarring, leading to cirrhosis and liver cancer. In a study of more than 6,000 people, those with the highest blood levels of vitamin D had a 40% lower risk of NAFLD. [11]

The optimal blood level of vitamin D

Yes, boosting your blood level of vitamin D should be a "priority," as Dr. Holick said. But opinions about the *best* blood level vary quite a bit.

Let's start at the low end—the level recommended by The Institute of Medicine, the panel of experts that sets the "recommended daily allowances" for individual nutrients used by the U.S. government.

In 2010, the Institute of Medicine reaffirmed its opinion that a "sufficient" blood level of vitamin D is 20 ng/ml (nanograms per milliliter).

"That's not the case," Dr. Holick told me. And he should know.

The Institute of Medicine created that level based on Dr. Holick's research from the 1990s, which showed that blood levels above 20 ng/ml did not affect levels of parathyroid hormone—a metabolic signal that the body has sufficient vitamin D. Yes, Dr. Holick said, levels below 20 ng/ml are a sign of a *severe deficiency* of vitamin D. But that doesn't mean levels just above 20 are sufficient for optimal health.

"There is now an abundance of evidence linking levels from 20 to 30 to *poor* health, including prediabetes and diabetes," Dr. Holick told me. Blood levels in the 20 to 30 range are not a sign of vitamin D *deficiency,* but of vitamin D *insufficiency*—and (as we mentioned earlier) the vast majority of Americans have insufficient levels of vitamin D.

Should you aim for 30 ng/ml?

Yes, says Dr. Holick. But many other health experts say you should aim higher. A *lot* higher.

40 ng/ml is the optimal level, I was told by William Grant, PhD, founder and director of the Sunlight, Nutrition and Health Research Center, in San Francisco, California, a non-profit devoted to research and education about the benefits of vitamin D.

45 to 60 ng/ml, said Mark Hyman, MD, chairman of the Institute for Functional Medicine and author of *The Blood Sugar Solution.*

50 to 80 ng/ml, says John Cannell, MD, the executive director of the Vitamin D Council and author of *The Athlete's Edge: Faster, Quicker and Stronger with Vitamin D.*

"This is the natural level normally achieved by people who work in the sun," he told me.

60 to 80 ng/ml, is the level she helps her clients with diabetes achieve, said Paula Vetter.

(Whatever level you choose, it's pretty clear the best level is *not* 20 ng/ml, as recommended by the Institute of Malnutrition. Oh, sorry, I meant to say, The Institute of Medicine…)

Personally, I opt for the highest range and encourage my health coaching clients to do the same.

That level is safe, experts agree. (More about the safety of vitamin D in a moment.)

And it's well worth achieving, said Dr. Cannell—because, along with diabetes, there are more than 125 conditions, disorders and diseases that you can prevent, control or reverse by increasing your blood levels of vitamin D.

Next question: How do you figure out your blood level of vitamin D? Simple: By taking a blood test.

Testing blood levels of vitamin D

Of course, you don't have to get your blood level of vitamin D tested. You can just implement a strategy for boosting vitamin D levels (discussed in the next section) and hope for the best.

But since having an optimal level of vitamin D is key to preventing prediabetes…or stopping prediabetes from turning into diabetes…or controlling diabetes and its complications…I think it's a smart move to discover and track your levels of vitamin D.

And it's not that hard. Or that expensive. In fact, it doesn't even have to involve a visit to the doctor.

Direct Labs. This company offers discounted blood tests directly to consumers. They charge $59 for a *25-hydroxyvitamin D test*—a test that would cost you $221 if your doctor ordered it. You order the test either online or by phone, and then go to a national laboratory service (like LabCorp) to have the blood drawn; the results are sent to you directly. (For ordering information, see the Resources section at the end of the chapter.)

Important: Make sure you order the *25-hydroxyvitamin D, or 25(OH)D, test* and not the *1,25-dihydroxyvitamin D test*, which is also offered at Direct Labs. The latter test does *not* accurately measure blood levels of vitamin D, but is sometimes incorrectly ordered (including by doctors).

ZRT Laboratory. You can order an at-home vitamin D blood test from ZRT Laboratory at the website of The Vitamin D Council and several other websites. (See the Resources section at the end of the chapter.)

You send for the test ($65 to $75)…you'll be sent the kit… you take a few blood samples with a device much like a finger-prick glucose monitor…you send in the samples…and you're sent the results.

Bruce Hollis, PhD, professor of Biochemistry and Molecular Biology at the Medical University of South Carolina, and one of the world's leading authorities on vitamin D testing, has reviewed the test and says it is accurate and reflects the "gold standard" of vitamin D testing, Dr.

Cannell told me. He recommends testing every six months.

www.grassrootshealth.com This is the website of The Grassroots Health D*Action Project, dedicated to solving the vitamin D deficiency epidemic. You order a ZRT Laboratory Test at the site for $65—and you also provide health data to be used as part of a study on vitamin D.

The 41 expert vitamin D researchers and medical practitioners who form the "Scientists Panel" of Grassroots Health recommend a blood level of 40 to 60 ng/ml—and say a daily intake of approximately 4,300 IU of vitamin D is necessary to achieve that level, if you start out at 20 ng/ml.

Is that a good recommendation for supplementation? Many experts think so…

The best supplement, the right dose

"I recommend supplementation at anywhere from 2,000 to 5,000 IU, depending on results from the blood test," says Vetter.

"I recommend you take vitamin D to optimize your level," said Dr. Hyman. "Most people require an additional 2,000 to 5,000 units of vitamin D3 a day."

Notice he said *Vitamin D3*, not Vitamin D2.

"I think *cholecalciferol*—vitamin D3—is the preferred form of oral vitamin D3, since it is the compound your skin makes naturally when you go out into the sun," Dr. Cannell said. "It is more potent and perhaps even safer than the synthetic analog, *ergocalciferol*—vitamin D2—that is found in many supplements.

(A recent study of 183 diabetes patients with vitamin D deficiency proves his point: treatment with vitamin D2 did *not* boost blood levels.) [12]

Dr. Cannell recommends 5,000 IU of vitamin D3 daily.

"Unless you're outdoors a lot or use a tanning booth, you need 5,000 IU a day to stay healthy," he said.

Why not get that amount in food? "To get that amount from D-fortified milk, for example, you'd need to drink 50 glasses a day," he said.

"Ingestion of 100 IU of vitamin D—a typical amount in a serving of D-fortified food—raises blood levels by only 1 ng/ml," Dr. Holick said.

A study that proves a supplement of 4,000 IU works to achieve higher levels of vitamin D was conducted at the Medical University of South Carolina. It involved 47 people, 65% with blood levels below 20 at the beginning of the study. A daily dose of 4,000 IU for one year brought the levels of every participant above 32 ng/ml. [13]

And taking 2,000 to 5,000 IU of vitamin D daily does *not* have to be expensive.

You can order reasonably priced and pharmaceutical-grade supplements of vitamin D—in 1,000, 2,000, 5,000 and 50,000 IU capsules—from Biotech Pharmacal. (See the Resources section at the end of the chapter for ordering information.)

For example, 100, 5,000 IU capsules cost $7.30—at a capsule a day, that's about $25 for a year's supply of vitamin D.

Vitamin D is very safe

Maybe you've heard or read that vitamin D builds up in the system and that taking too much can cause an overdose. Is 2,000 to 5,000 IU of daily vitamin D *dangerous*? No, says Dr. Cannell.

"There is not a single case in the medical literature of vitamin D toxicity while taking regular, daily doses of 25,000 IU or less," he told me.

"Scientists use a term called the *therapeutic index* to calculate toxicity—the dose of a normal substance that would be toxic," he continued. "Water, for example, has a therapeutic index of ten—if you drink eight, eight-ounce glasses of water you're fine, but if you drink eighty, you die. Vitamin D, in comparison, has a therapeutic index of twenty—it's literally safer than water! Worrying about vitamin D toxicity is like worrying about drowning when you're dying of thirst."

But there are two ways you *can* drown in vitamin D. Blood levels of vitamin D are unsafe if they exceed 100 ng/ml. (Another reason to track your blood levels if you supplement with high doses.) And if you have a *granulomatous disorder* (a range of disorders in which a dense collection of inflammatory cells called a *granuloma* are formed) you are potentially hypersensitive to vitamin D and shouldn't take the supplement.

Let the sunshine in

Sunlight is nature's way of creating vitamin D in your body—and as we all know, it's not nice to fool Mother Nature. "Exposing bare skin to sunlight from late spring to early fall, when the rays of the sun are most direct, is the best way to boost your blood levels of vitamin D," Dr. Holick said. And bare means bare of sunscreen, too. (However, always use sunscreen on your face to avoid wrinkling.)

His advice:

During the months of May to October…any time between 10 am and 3pm…on two to three days a week…expose your arms and legs (54% of your total skin surface) to sunlight.

How much sunlight?

"It varies quite a bit from person to person, depending on skin type—from redheads with fair skin that always burns, to people of African origin who never burn," Dr. Holick said.

Dr. Holick's recommendation for getting the amount of sunshine that's just right for you: Know how long it takes to get a mild sunburn on your face—and then expose your no-sunscreen arms and legs for 30 to 50% of that time, following the above guidelines for time of year, time of day, and days of the week. For example, if it takes half an hour of sun exposure to be pink, expose your arms and legs for no more than 15 minutes before applying sunscreen to them.

Anti-diabetes secrets in the next chapter...

- The sad, dark secret of diabetes: four out of five people with the disease are also depressed—increasing their risk of death by 50%!

- Why antidepressants *don't* work for four out of five people with depression.

- The depression-beating, mood-boosting power of fish oil supplements—but *only* if you take a supplement with the right combination and amount of the fatty acids EPA and DHA.

EXPERTS AND CONTRIBUTORS:

John Cannell, MD, is the executive director of the Vitamin D Council, in San Luis Obispo, California, whose mission is to educate the general public and health professionals on vitamin D, sun exposure, and the vitamin D deficiency pandemic.
Website: www.vitamindcouncil.org

William Grant, PhD, is the founder and director of the Sunlight, Nutrition and Health Research Center, in San Francisco, California, a non-profit devoted to research and education about the benefits of vitamin D.
Website: www.sunarc.org

Michael Holick, MD, PhD, is a professor of medicine, physiology and biophysics at Boston University Medical Center (BUMC), and the BUMC director of the General Clinic Research Unit, the Bone Health Clinic, and the Heliotherapy Light and Skin Research Center. He is the author more than 300 research articles, and the book *The Vitamin D Solution: A 3-Step Strategy to Cure Our Most Common Health Problem.*

Mark Hyman, MD, was co-medical director of Canyon Ranch for almost 10 years and is now the chairman of the Institute for Functional Medicine and founder and medical director of the UltraWellness Center. He is the *New York Times* bestselling author of *UltraMetabolism, The UltraMind Solution,* and the *UltraSimple Diet.*
Websites: www.drhyman.com, www.bloodsugarsolution.com
Facebook: facebook.com/drmarkhyman
Twitter: @markhymanmd

Paula Vetter, RN, is a holistic family nurse practitioner, certified herbalist, certified diabetes educator, Reiki Master/teacher, certified EFT practitioner, and personal wellness coach.
Website: www.profoundwellness.com
Phone: **(330) 815-0340**

RESOURCES:

For a discounted, reliable vitamin D blood test you can order directly via the internet:
Direct Labs
Website: www.directlabs.com
Phone: 1-800-908-0000

For a "gold standard," at-home vitamin D blood test from ZRT Laboratory:
www.vitamindcouncil.org
www.grassrootshealth.org
www.zrtlab.com

To order inexpensive, pharmaceutical-grade vitamin D supplements:
BioTech Pharmacal
Website: www.biotechpharmacal.com

REFERENCES:

1. Holick MF. D-iabetes and D-eath D-efying vitamin D. *Nature Reviews/Endocrinology*, July 2012, 8, 388-390.

2. Gagnon C, et al. Low serum 25-hydroxvitamin D is associated with increased risk of the development of the metabolic syndrome at five years: results from a national, population-based prospective study. *Journal of Clinical Endocrinology and Metabolism*, 2012 Jun;97(6):1953-61

3. Deleskog A, et al. Low serum 25-hydroxvitamin D level predicts progression to type 2 diabetes in individuals with prediabetes but not with normal glucose tolerance. *Diabetologia,* 2012 Jun;55(6):1668-78.

4. Thomas G, et al. Vitamin D levels predict all-cause and cardiovascular disease mortality in subjects with the metabolic syndrome: the Ludwigshafen Risk and Cardiovascular Health Study. *Diabetes Care*, 2012 May;35(5):1158-64.

5. Reis JP, et al. Vitamin D status and cardiometabolic risk factors in the United States Adolescent Population. *Pediatrics*, 2009 Sep;124(3).

6. Talaei A, et al. The effect of vitamin D on insulin resistance in patients with type 2 diabetes. *Diabetology & Metabolic Syndrome*, 2013 Feb 26;5(1):8.

7. Al-Daghri NM, et al. Vitamin D supplementation as an adjuvant therapy for patients with TD2M: an 18-month prospective interventional study. *Cardiovascular Diabetology*, 2012 July 18:11(1):85.

8. Bell, DS. Reversal of the Symptoms of Diabetic Neuropathy through Correction of Vitamin D Deficiency in a Type 1 Diabetic Patient. *Case Reports in Endocrinology*, 2012;20912:16506. Epub 20-12 Dec 12.

9. Shehab D, et al. Does Vitamin D deficiency play a role in peripheral neuropathy in Type 2 Diabetes? *Diabetes Medicine*, 2012 Jan;29(1):43-9.

10. Huang Y, et al. Oral supplementation with cholecalciferol 800 IU ameliorates albuminuria in Chinese type 2 diabetic patients with nephropathy. *PLOS ONE*, 2012;7(11):e50510.

11. Rhee EJ, et al. High serum vitamin D levels reduce the risk of nonalcoholic fatty liver disease in healthy men independent of the metabolic syndrome. *Journal of Endocrinology*, 2013 Feb 13.

12. Alshayeb HM, et al. Chronic Kidney Disease and Diabetes Mellitus Predict Resistance to Vitamin D Replacement Therapy. *American Journal of Medicine and Science*, 2012 Dec 5. [Epub ahead of print]

13. Garrett-Mayer E, et al. Vitamin D3 supplementation (4000 IU/d for 1 y) eliminates differences in circulating 25-hydroxyvitamin D between African-American and white men. *American Journal of Clinical Nutrition*, 2012 Aug;96(2):332-6.

Chapter 13

Omega-3

Depression raises the death risk from diabetes by 50%.
The happy remedy: Omega-3.

Depression is like living in a hole.

You feel sad or empty inside—most of the day, nearly every day. You can't find any pleasure in everyday activities you used to enjoy. Your concentration is shot and you can't think clearly. You feel worthless or guilty. You may even think about turning that hole into your grave.

With other symptoms of depression you're either stuck in the hole—or running around it in circles. You have no appetite—or binge. You're slow as a slug—or hyperactive. You sleep 10 hours a day—or hardly sleep.

If you've got most of the symptoms just mentioned, you have what doctors call "severe" depression. If you have five or less, you've got the "moderate" or "mild" version. Either way, those symptoms can stick around for weeks or months.

Depression itself is bad enough. But it has a secret physical cost most people don't know about.

Depression doubles the risk of developing diabetes.

Given the fact that depression can lead to diabetes, it's no surprise that depression and diabetes are often found together. In fact, having diabetes doubles your risk of being depressed! It's estimated that 40 to 50% of people with diabetes suffer from depression.

And that blue mood darkens just about every aspect of the disease.

If you're diagnosed with diabetes *and* depression (as compared to just diabetes), you're also likely to have…

- **Higher A1C,** a measurement of long-term blood sugar levels. [1]

- **Triple the risk of heart disease,** the illness that kills most people with diabetes. [2]

- **Nearly three times the level of C-reactive protein,** a biomarker of chronic inflammation—and inflammation not only fuels diabetes but other chronic diseases, like heart disease, cancer and Alzheimer's. [2]

- **16% higher levels of cortisol,** the stress hormone that spikes blood sugar levels. [2]

- **41% greater chance of being hospitalized for diabetes-related problems.** [3]

- **50% higher risk of dying**—a shocking statistic, from a 2013 study involving more than 42,000 people with diabetes. [4]

Why does depression both cause and worsen diabetes?

"The underlying mechanisms are still unclear," said researchers from the Department of Psychiatry at the University of Illinois, in a paper in *Neuropsychopharmacology*. [5]

But experts do know that depression—for whatever reason—batters the body. Scientists with the World Health Organization say it's the "leading cause of disability" and the "leading cause of disease burden" in the world. (For example, in an analysis of 28 studies on heart disease, researchers discovered depression was *the most important risk factor* for developing the disease.)

But there's a simple solution to depression, right? Just get in line for one of the 170 million prescriptions for antidepressants that American doctors write every year.

Well, don't rush off to the pharmacy just yet. There's a big problem with antidepressants, even if you overlook common side effects like digestive upset, headaches, weight gain and sexual dysfunction.

The drugs don't work.

Antidepressants: no more effective than a placebo

That's the conclusion of a study in the *Journal of the American Medical Association*, which I first reported in my book *Breakthroughs in Natural Healing 2011*.

In the study, researchers at the University of Pennsylvania analyzed data from six other studies on antidepressants, involving more than 700 depressed people. The benefits of taking the drug? How about "nonexistent"…

"True drug effects—an advantage of antidepressant medications over placebo—were nonexistent to negligible among depressed patients with mild, moderate or even severe baseline symptoms," said Jay C. Fournier, PhD, the study leader. (The antidepressants *did* work for people with "very severe" symptoms, he said.)

And here's the kicker: four out of five people who are depressed have mild to moderate depression. So antidepressants don't work any better than a placebo for 80% of the people who take them!

Dr. Fournier noted that most of the previous studies "proving" antidepressants work involved only patients with severe depression—a fact that most doctors and patients probably don't know. (And drug companies never mention.)

"What this and other studies show is that the majority of people on antidepressants—the four out of five people with mild or moderate depression—are essentially taking an expensive placebo with nasty side effects, such as weight gain and lowered libido," I was told by Stephen Ilardi, PhD, associate professor of clinical psychology at the University of Kansas, and author of *The Depression Cure: The 6-Step Program to Beat Depression Without Drugs*.

Omega-3 treats depression—for real

Fortunately, there are two *nutrients* that dozens of studies show *can* treat (or prevent) depression:

EPA (eicosapentaenoic acid) and DHA (docosahexaenoic acid), the omega-3 fatty acids found in fatty fish such as salmon, tuna, sardines and mackerel, and in fish oil supplements.

"The evidence for omega-3 in the treatment of depression is substantial," I was told by Carol Locke, MD, a psychiatrist in Lincoln, Massachusetts, former faculty member in the Department of Psychiatry at Harvard Medical School, co-founder and director of the Center for Creating Health in California—and co-author of one of the first scientific papers looking at the depression-taming power of omega-3.

Let's take a look at some of that evidence…

Lower levels of omega-3 in depressed people. In a review of 14 studies, researchers from Taiwan found depressed people had "significantly lower" bodily levels of EPA and DHA compared to people who weren't depressed. [6] "Our findings provide…a rationale for using Omega-3 fatty acids as an alternative treatment for depression," concluded the researchers.

Eat more fish, suffer less depression. In a four-year study of more than 10,000 people, researchers found that people with the highest intake of EPA and DHA from fish had the fewest "depressive symptoms." [7]

"A significant antidepressant effect of Omega-3." In a review of 10 studies on omega-3 and depression, omega-3 supplements improved depressive symptoms 61% better than placebo, reported researchers in the *Journal of Clinical Psychiatry*. [8]

Eases depression during menopause. Menopause doubles the risk of depression. Researchers from Harvard Medical School gave two grams of omega-3 daily to women in the "menopausal transition" who were depressed—and their level of depression dropped 56% in two months. They had fewer hot flashes, too. [9]

Better moods for seniors with the blues. All too often, the golden years are tinged with the blues. In a study of 66 people aged 65 and older, taking one gram of omega-3 daily for six months helped relieve mild-to-moderate depression. [10]

When antidepressants don't work, antidepressants *and* omega-3 do. Seventy people with "treatment-resistant" depression had an EPA supplement added to their antidepressant regimen. 53% of those taking the supplement had a significant improvement in their depression—compared to only 29% of patients who didn't take the EPA. [11]

Works for bipolar depression, too. Australian researchers analyzed five studies that treated bipolar disorder (manic-depression) with omega-3 supplements and found "strong evidence that bipolar disorder depressive symptoms may be improved" by omega-3. [12]

Help after depression. Bouts of depression don't last forever—can omega-3 help *after* you've recovered from depression? Yes, say Dutch scientists, who found that four weeks of omega-3 supplements improved decision-making, tension levels and mood in "recovered depressed individuals." [13] In another study, higher blood levels of omega-3s were linked to better memory in seniors who had previously been depressed. [14]

All that evidence and more led the American Psychiatric Association to conclude that an omega-3 supplement of 1 to 3 grams may be useful in treating depression. (And to recommend that everyone—depressed or not—eat fish three times a week.)

Omega-3 for depression in diabetes

Okay, omega-3 works to ease depression. But could it work to ease depression associated with diabetes? Yes, according to a group of Dutch scientists writing in the journal *Diabetic Medicine.*

"Supplementation with omega-3—in particular EPA—may be a safe and helpful tool to reduce the incidence of depression and to treat depression in Type 2 diabetes," they concluded after an extensive review of the scientific literature on omega-3, depression and diabetes.

"I frequently recommend an omega-3 supplement for my patients with type 2 diabetes, especially if they suffer from depression," I was told by Jennifer Warren, MD, director of the Physicians Healthy Weight Center in Hampton, New Hampshire.

How Omega-3 works

Why are omega-3 fatty acids such powerful *natural* antidepressants ? Because they feed your brain. Without enough omega-3…

- The outer covering of brains cells (*neurons*) degenerates.

- Neurons generate less *serotonin*, a neurotransmitter that helps control mood.

- The cellular receptors for *dopamine*—another neurotransmitter linked to mood—become malformed.

- *Dendrites*—the branching extensions that channel messages into and out of the cell—have fewer branches.

- There are fewer *synapses*, the bridges between cells.

In other words, an omega-3 deficiency is a sad story for your brain cells—and for your mood.

But not all omega-3 supplements are equally good at nourishing your brain and banishing the blues.

The best supplement for depression: higher in EPA than DHA

In an analysis of 15 studies involving nearly 1,000 people, researchers found that supplements with 60% or more of their omega-3 from EPA were the most effective in relieving depression ("Supplements with EPA less than 60% were ineffective," said the scientists.) They also found that for the omega-3 to work, the supplement's dose of EPA had to be 200 to 2,200 milligrams more than the dose of DHA. [15]

And when scientists tested EPA against DHA—with one group of depressed patients taking EPA and another taking DHA—only the group taking EPA had an improvement in their symptoms. [16]

An omega-3 supplement designed to beat depression

One supplement with just that combination is OmegaBrite, which was specifically formulated to supply the quantity of EPA that can combat depression, said Dr. Locke, who is the founder and CEO of OmegaBrite.

There's a lot that I like about OmegaBrite, a supplement I often talk about with my health coaching clients who struggle with low moods, anxiety or other types of emotional stress.

It has an EPA/DHA ratio of 7:1 EPA, with 350 mg of EPA and 50 mg of DHA per capsule. (And the soft gel capsules are small and easy to swallow.)

Consumerlab.com (which identifies the best nutritional products through independent testing) gave the product its seal of approval, verifying that it's pure and potent, and that its labeling accurately reflects what's in the supplement.

The product is "pharmaceutical-grade"—in fact, Dr. Locke coined that term, which is now widely used among manufacturers of nutritional supplements to indicate purity and potency.

And what *makes* OmegaBrite pharmaceutical-grade is that it undergoes several steps of distillation that remove all heavy metals and toxins (and fishy aftertaste). It's also manufactured with a patented process that prevents oxidation of the fatty acids. And every batch or "lot" of the product is independently tested at a certified lab to verify purity, quality and label claims.

How much OmegaBrite do you need to prevent or treat depression?

For maintaining a positive mood even if you're not depressed, Dr. Locke recommends three to four capsules a day. "A lot of people who don't consider themselves depressed feel better on four a day," she told me. ("Always take the supplement with food to maximize absorption," she added.)

For mild to moderate depression, she recommends four to six capsules a day. If you have severe depression or bipolar disorder, she recommends six to eight.

(Needless to say, always talk to your health care professional about the supplements you're taking.)

And those recommendations work…

"I feel the best I have felt in a long time."

"I have been diagnosed with thyroid disease, type 2 diabetes, and have had a bout or two of depression," said Jenn A. "I need to say that, after taking OmegaBrite, I feel the best that I have felt in a long time. As the winter approaches, and the usual anxiety of the holidays rushes in, I find myself smiling and laughing things off more. I only wish that I had known about OmegaBrite sooner."

"I had heart disease, type 2 diabetes, arthritis, and bipolar disorder," said David R. "In the last six months I have been on a diet rich in omega-3, including 6 capsules of OmegaBrite everyday—and my life has changed in every way. I am no longer arthritic or bipolar, I have a healthy heart—and two weeks ago my physician was astonished to say that the results of a

<u>hemoglobin test confirmed I am no longer diabetic</u>. I can honestly say I would not be alive and healthy if it was not for OmegaBrite."

To buy OmegaBrite, see the ordering information in the Resources section at the end of the chapter.

Dousing the disease-feeding fire of chronic inflammation

Omega-3 fatty acids are *anti-inflammatory*. And that may be one of the reasons why they prevent, control and reverse depression—and many other chronic problems that plague diabetes patients, like heart disease.

"Chronic inflammation is the common denominator underlying many widespread diseases in the industrialized world—diabetes, atherosclerosis, Alzheimer's disease, heart disease, allergies, asthma, stroke, metabolic syndrome, and even many types of cancer," said Dr. Ilardi.

"Inflammation is also one of the big culprits behind the depression epidemic," he continued. "Over time, it interferes with the brain's ability to manufacture and use serotonin, and it can lead to reduced activity in the frontal cortex. It also impairs the function of brain regions such as the *hippocampus*—critical for memory function—that have been implicated in the onset of depression. Finally, chronic inflammation causes the brain to ramp up its stress response in an attempt to put things back in balance, since the stress hormone *cortisol* has powerful anti-inflammatory properties. Unfortunately, cortisol has its own set of depressive effects on the brain."

Dr. Ilardi recommends a starting omega-3 dose of 1000 milligrams of EPA and 500 milligrams of DHA for all of his patients. "If you currently have symptoms of depression, or if you want to help prevent the onset of illness in the future, this is the dose I suggest you begin with," he said. If you're on a tight budget, he recommends Mega EFA (800 mg EPA, 400 mg DHA) from Neutraceutical Sciences Institute, available online at www.vitacost.com.

Another brand of fish oil supplement often recommended to me by health professionals I interview is Nordic Naturals. For depression, consider either EPA (850 EPA, 250 DHA) or EPA Xtra (1060 EPA, 274 DHA). (www.nordicnaturals.com)

Anti-diabetes secrets in the next chapter...

- Drugs don't work well for diabetic nerve pain—but alpha-lipoic acid nutrient does!

- His foot ulcers and poor eyesight led his conventional doctors to predict amputation and blindness—but alpha-lipoic acid reversed his diabetic complications in just *three weeks*. The amazing story.

- The science-proven alpha-lipoic regimen for relieving neuropathic pain.

EXPERTS AND CONTRIBUTORS:

Stephen Ilardi, PhD, is an associate professor of clinical psychology at the University of Kansas, and author of *The Depression Cure: The 6-Step Program to Beat Depression Without Drugs*.

Carol Locke, MD, is a psychiatrist in Lincoln, Massachusetts and a former faculty member in the Department of Psychiatry at Harvard Medical School.

Jennifer Warren, MD, is the director of the Physicians Healthy Weight Center in Hampton, New Hampshire.

RESOURCES:

To order OmegaBrite, an omega-3 supplement specifically formulated to prevent and treat depression:
Website: www.omegabrite.com
Call: 800-383-2030
Email: updates@OmegaBrite.com

REFERENCES:

1. Bot M, et al. Differential associations between depressive symptoms and glycaemic control in outpatients with diabetes. *Diabetes Medicine*, 2013 Mar;30(3):e115-22.

2. Alvarez A, et al. Endocrine and inflammatory profiles in type 2 diabetic patients with and without major depressive disorder. *BMC Research Notes*, 2013 Feb 14;6(1):61.

3. Davydow DS, et al. Depression and Risk of Hospitalizations for Ambulatory Care-Sensitive Conditions in Patients with Diabetes. *Journal of General Internal Medicine*, 2013 Jan 17. [Epub ahead of print]

4. Park M, et al. Depression and risk of mortality in individuals with diabetes: a meta-analysis. *General Hospital Psychiatry*, 2013 Feb 12. [Epub ahead of print]

5. Zhang A, et al. White Matter Tract Integrity of Anterior limb of Internal Capsule in Major Depression and Type 2 Diabetes. *Neuropsychopharmacology*, 2013 Feb 6. [Epub ahead of print]

6. Lin PY, et al. A meta-analytic review of polyunsaturated fatty acid compositions in patients with depression. *Biological Psychiatry*, 2010 Jul 15;68(2):140-7.

7. Hoffmire CA, et al. Associations between omega-3 poly-unsaturated fatty acids from fish consumption and severity of depressive symptoms: an analysis of the 2005-2008 National Health and Nutrition Examination Survey. *Prostaglandins, Leukotrienes & Essential Fatty Acids*, 2012 Apr;86(4-5):155-60.

8. Lin PY, et al. A meta-analytic review of double-blind, placebo-controlled trials of antidepressant efficacy of omega-3 fatty acids. *Journal of Clinical Psychiatry*, 2007 Jul;68(7):1056-61.

9. Freeman MP, et al. Omega-3 fatty acids for major depressive disorder associated with the menopausal transition: a preliminary open trial. *Menopause*, 2011 Mar;18(3):279-84.

10. Tajalizadekhoob Y, et al. The effect of low-dose omega 3 fatty acids on the treatment of mild to moderate depression in the elderly: a double-blind, randomized, placebo-controlled study. *European Archives of Psychiatry and Clinical Neuroscience*, 2011 Dec;261(80);539-49.

11. Peet M, et al. A dose-ranging study of the effects of ethyl-eicosapentaenoate in patients with ongoing depression despite apparently adequate treatment with standard drugs. *Archives of General Psychiatry*, 2002; 59: 913-919.

12. Sarris J, et al. Omega-3 for bipolar disorder: meta-analyses of use in mania and bipolar depression. *Journal of Clinical Psychiatry*, 2012 Jan;73(1):81-6.

13. Antypa N, et al. Effects of omega-3 fatty acid supplementation on mood and emotional information processing in recovered depressed individuals. *Journal of Psychopharmacology*, 2012 Jay;26(5):738-43.

14. Chiu CC, et al. Associations between n-3 PUFA concentrations and cognitive function after recovery from late-life depression.

15. Sublette ME, et al. Meta-analysis: Effects of Eicosapentaenoic Acid in Clinical Trials in Depression. *Journal of Clinical Psychiatry,* 2011 December; 72(12): 1577-1584.

16. Mozaffari-Kosravi H, et al. Eicosapentaenoic acid versus docosahexaenoic acid in mild-to-moderate depression: A randomized, double-blind, placebo-controlled trial. *European Neuropsychopharmacology*, 2012 Aug 8 [Epub ahead of print]

Chapter 14

Alpha Lipoic Acid

Natural relief for nerve pain

Mr. Michaels, a 60-year-old diabetes patient, was in bad shape. His eyesight was failing. He had been diagnosed with heart disease. But worst of all were his *feet*. They hurt. They *burned*.

The problem: Diabetic peripheral neuropathy—damage to the nerves of the feet (and sometimes the hands).

Your toes and feet can hurt…or burn…or tingle, with electric-like shocks…or cramp…or be so numb it's hard to find your footing. Sometimes the problem becomes so bad you can't even walk.

After five years with diabetes, 20% of patients are hobbled by peripheral neuropathy. After ten years, the rate is 40%.

And that's just what was happening to Mr. Michaels. The soles of his feet burned as if they were being held to an invisible fire. And no firefighters were on the way…

His doctor had told him there were no medications that could help—the pain would worsen, and eventually his toes and feet might have to be amputated. His eye doctor told him that he had *diabetic retinopathy*—damage to the retina at the back of the eye; his eyesight would worsen and he might go blind.

So, with nothing to lose, Mr. Michaels made an appointment with Burt Berkson, MD, PhD, the medical director of the Integrative Medical Center of New Mexico, in Las Cruces. For several decades, Dr. Berkson had been the FDA's principle investigator for the use of alpha lipoic acid as a drug, and he is the author of *The Alpha Lipoic Acid Breakthrough*.

Dr. Berkson examined Mr. Michaels and prescribed alpha lipoic acid: 300 milligrams (mg), three times a day. The results were remarkable—and rapid.

"After three weeks, the constant burning in the soles of his feet disappeared," Dr. Berkson told me. "He also noticed that he was able to read without his glasses."

How can *one* supplement—alpha lipoic acid—make such a huge difference?

<u>Because alpha lipoic acid is a super-antioxidant.</u>

It smothers the oxidation (and resulting inflammation) that slowly but surely destroys tiny blood vessels (microcirculation)—the type of destruction that eventually results in complications like neuropathy and retinopathy.

Let's look more closely at the power of alpha lipoic acid (which I'll abbreviate as ALA throughout the rest of this chapter) to defeat the complications of diabetes—particularly peripheral neuropathy.

Alpha lipoic acid: a close look at a super-antioxidant

In their recent scientific paper, *Diabetes and alpha lipoic acid*, [1] a team of researchers from the University of British Columbia describe all the ways ALA works to "manage diabetic complications," with its "clearest benefit…in patients with diabetic neuropathy."

"ALA," they write, (take a deep breath; this will be over soon) "acts as a cofactor for pyruvate dehydrogenase and an alpha-ketoglutarate dehydrogenase activity, and is also required for the oxidative decarboxylation of pyruvate to acetyl-CoA, a critical step bridging glycolysis and the citric acid cycle."

Allow me to translate…

ALA is manufactured in the *mitochondria,* the tiny energy factories in every cell. Without it, your body can't turn food into energy—it's *that* basic to life and health.

Given in supplement-sized doses of 100 mg or more, ALA can…

Squelch *reactive oxygen species*, the oxidants (aka, *free radicals*) that mug other molecules, stealing their electrons and doing a lot of cellular damage in the process. This *oxidative stress* causes constant, low-level systemic inflammation as the immune system rallies to repair cellular damage. It is the driving force behind most chronic diseases, including diabetes.

And not only is ALA a super-powerful antioxidant; it's also an ambidextrous one. Most antioxidants are either water-soluble (like vitamin C) or fat-soluble (like vitamin E). ALA is unique because it's both. What are the benefits of this odd property? Water-soluble vitamins stop oxidation *inside* the cell, where the environment is watery, while fat-soluble vitamins stop oxidation *outside* the cell, which has a fatty surface or "skin." ALA uniquely stops oxidation inside AND out.

Stop other antioxidants from turning into pro-oxidants. You probably think of the antioxidants vitamins C and E as good guys, without an evil bone in their molecular bodies. But they can be like cops who become corrupted: after they're done with their *anti-* work, they turn into *pro-*oxidants—the same type of free radicals they were arresting a nanosecond ago.

Super-antioxidant ALA stops the good guys from going bad. Then it even regenerates them, turning them back into fully functioning antioxidants.

And ALA itself is the ultimate good guy: unlike vitamins C and E, it never becomes a free radical.

Boosts glutathione, another super-antioxidant. ALA is your body's super-antioxidant, but there's another, little-known superhero in the neighborhood: *glutathione*. Glutathione disarms free radicals, protects proteins from oxidation, detoxifies pollutants and revs up the immune system—and ALA helps the body make a whole lot more of it. And just as it does with vitamins C and E, ALA also stops glutathione from turning traitor and becoming a pro-oxidant.

Tames copper and iron. High levels of these metals trigger oxidation. (In fact, some health experts think that excess copper from drinking water and multivitamin/mineral supplements is a main cause of the oxidation in the brain that leads to Alzheimer's disease.) ALA neutralizes them.

Blocks nuclear factor kappa beta (NFKB)—the primal trigger of inflammation. Found in every cell, *nuclear factor kappa beta* is a protein with a lot of responsibilities—it passes the informational baton from DNA to RNA, so your cells know what to do. Among its many roles, it helps your immune system defend cells from free radicals, viruses and other troublemakers. However, NFKB can easily *overreact*, producing immune-caused inflammation.

ALA helps keep it calm.

Turns on AMPK (AMP-activated protein kinase)—just like diabetes drugs. AMPK is an enzyme that improves the output of insulin (the hormone that ushers glucose out of the bloodstream and into cells)…helps muscles use glucose…burns fat…and also blocks the overproduction of fat. (AMPK is a target of several diabetes drugs.)

More ALA=more AMPK.

Bottom line: ALA's "antioxidant effects may be particularly useful in slowing the development of diabetic complications such as diabetic neuropathy," conclude the researchers. And they cite eight studies on diabetic peripheral neuropathy to prove their point. Let's take a quick look at some of that research…

Big studies, positive results

A recent scientific study on ALA for diabetic neuropathy analyzed the results of all the best studies to date—a so-called *meta-analysis*. [2]

First, the Dutch researchers noted that the medications typically used for neuropathy—antidepressants, antiepileptics and opioids—"are limited in their effectiveness, they have considerable side effects," and they do nothing to address the high blood sugar and inflammation that cause neuropathy.

Having said that about the drugs, the researchers then present their analysis of the four best studies on using ALA—involving more than 600 diabetes patients, who received the nutrient either intravenously or as dietary supplement, at levels ranging from 600 to 1800 mg daily.

Doctors measure the severity of neuropathy using a "Total Symptom Score" test that evaluates the degree of pain, burning, numbness and the strange, uncomfortable tingling and itching sensations called *paresthesia*.

A significant improvement—an average 50% reduction in all these symptoms—was reported in all the studies.

The most effective dose was 600 mg. daily—delivered either intravenously or by supplement. Higher doses didn't produce faster or better relief.

And the researchers noted that the effect of ALA on neuropathic pain was "unexpectedly rapid"—relief was achieved after only three to five weeks of treatment.

Treating thousands of diabetes patients over 35 years—with ALA

Those results aren't a surprise to Dr. Berkson. In our fascinating interview, he told me that doctors have been using ALA intravenously for diabetes since the 1970s, with one expert calling it "the wonder drug for reversal of diabetic complications." (ALA has been used as a "wonder drug" for many other health problems, including cardiovascular disease, cancer and liver disease, each of which merits its own chapter in Dr. Berkson's book on ALA.)

Over the past 35 years, Dr. Berkson has used ALA to treat thousands of patients with diabetic neuropathy, like Mr. Michaels. While we were on the phone, he described another dramatic case history:

"A very rich and prominent individual had been treated for his diabetic complications at one of the big, prestigious universities on the East Coast—with no success. He had severe neuropathy and was confined to a wheelchair. He also had severe retinopathy and wasn't able to read.

"One of his physicians told him about me, and he came out here with his entire entourage—bodyguards, cooks, the whole crew—and they rented 10 limousines and several condos. He stayed for three months, first receiving intravenous and then oral ALA. I also put him on a healthy diet, rich in leafy green vegetables, complex carbohydrates and non-processed proteins.

"After three months he was able to walk and read—a remarkable reversal of his complications."

The ideal ALA regimen

Most of Dr. Berkson's patients with diabetic peripheral neuropathy are given a regimen much like the tycoon's, starting with daily intravenous treatment with ALA (600 mg, twice a day).

Scientific research and his own clinical experience shows that three to five weeks of IV treatment are ideal for reversing diabetic neuropathy. But since most of the patients can only stay for a week or two, he advises them to find a nearby doctor who is a member of the American College for the Advancement of Medicine (ACAM), an organization of integrative-minded physicians that has invited him to numerous lectures and workshops to train its members in the use of intravenous alpha lipoic acid.

"Patients often travel out to see us, stay a week or two, we work out a protocol for them, and then their ACAM doctor continues it when they go home," he told me.

You can find an ACAM doctor near you either via the "Physician+Link" service on their website, www.acam.org, or by calling 1-800-532-3688.

After the intravenous treatment ends, his patients typically use a daily maintenance dose of 900 mg of supplemental ALA: 600 mg with one meal, and 300 mg with another.

He also advises patients to take a daily B-complex supplement when they take ALA, since the powerful antioxidant burns up B-vitamins as it does its work.

How safe is ALA? "I've been using it with patients for more than three decades and I've never seen any ill effects," he told me.

However, he said, you need to be cautious about the *type* of ALA you use. "Some of the Asian-sourced brands are industrial-grade, with impurities that may cause side effects."

He uses an ALA supplement (Lipoic 300) and a B-complex supplement (B-Stress) from the company Bio-Tech Pharmacal, which he says manufactures pharmaceutical-grade products that deliver the amount specified on the label. (This supplement company often receives glowing endorsements from clinicians I interview for my books. For ordering information, see the "Resources" section at the end of the chapter.) He also trusts and uses products from the supplement company Metabolic Maintenance. (See the "Resources" section for ordering info.)

Studies show a regimen starting with intravenous ALA and switching to oral ALA after three to five weeks is most effective for treating diabetic neuropathy. But, like Mr. Michaels, many diabetes patients have found relief by purchasing and using a supplement of ALA—and that's certainly a good place to start. If two months of 600 to 900 mg a day of oral ALA doesn't provide enough relief, you can investigate receiving intravenous ALA.

Dr. Berkson also advises his diabetes patients to take a high-dose multivitamin-mineral supplement (without iron), vitamin C (1,000 to 2,000 mg daily), selenium (200 micrograms daily), fish oil (he recommends Pro-Omega, from Nordic Naturals), vitamin D3 (1500 to 3000 IU daily), and chromium picolinate (200 mcg per meal).

For those with diabetic retinopathy, he adds the retina-protecting antioxidant *lutein* and the eye-strengthening herb *bilberry*.

"I think if a person with diabetes gets on a good diet, and a good exercise program, with regular aerobic exercise and weight-lifting, and takes the correct supplements, they can reverse their disease without drugs," he told me.

Worldwide praise for ALA

I searched the web to find out if diabetes patients were talking to each other about the power of ALA to heal diabetic neuropathy. They certainly were. A few examples…

ALA replaces a "worthless" neuropathy drug. "Right now, for my diabetes, I am taking 1200 mg of alpha lipoic acid," read a post at www.survivalistboards.com. "It has (knock wood) minimized my neuropathic burning of the feet, as well as some numbness of the fingers. I suspect it's also lowered my sugars. With my MD's approval, I replaced Januvia [for blood sugar control] with ALA and got rid of worthless (to me) Lyrica [for neuropathic pain]."

Not a skeptic now. "I am newly diagnosed, and my doctor sent me to a diabetes education class," said a post at http://forum.americandiabeteswholesale.com. "The doctor who led the class told us about alpha lipoic acid. He recommended 300 mg, twice a day, for six to eight weeks, to reverse neuropathy, and then 100 mg a day afterward. I was skeptical, but I have had neuropathy for several years, and the pain was becoming quite intense. I have been on this regimen for 3 weeks now—and I am already noticing a reduction in pain."

ALA "took care of it." "I had diabetes-induced neuropathy in my left hand only, never in my feet," says a post at www.diabetesdaily.com. "Had it for months. Getting my sugars down and taking alpha lipoic acid took care of it."

No side effects. I have type 2 diabetes, but control it without drugs, using diet and supplements," says a post at www.mombu.com. I use the super-antioxidant alpha lipoic acid, 200 mg, 4 times a day, for dealing with my neuropathy complications. No side effects that I am aware of, but check with your MD."

Thank you for telling me about ALA. "For my diabetic husband, lowering his blood sugar does not help the neuropathy," says a post at http://csn.cancer.org. "But as long as he takes 600 mg of alpha lipoic acid every day, the neuropathy is better controlled. And thank you again to the person who brought this to my attention a couple of years ago."

Anti-diabetes secrets in the next chapter...

- Why the insulin-producing "beta-cells" of your pancreas are burnt out like an overworked employee—and how coenzyme Q10 can restore their energy and performance.

- The reasons why you're probably *deficient* in coenzyme Q10.

- The many anti-diabetes benefits of coenzyme Q10—including better blood sugar control… preventing and reversing nerve pain…and protecting your heart, the main target of diabetic damage.

- Why cholesterol-lowering statin drugs *obliterate* coenzyme Q10—and what you must do to protect yourself if you're taking a statin.

EXPERTS AND CONTRIBUTORS:

Bert Berkson, MD, PhD, practices integrative medicine in Las Cruces, New Mexico, and is an adjunct professor at New Mexico State University. He is an expert consultant on alpha lipoic acid at the Centers for Disease Control. He is the author of several books on health and healing, including *The Alpha Lipoic Acid Breakthrough.*
Website: www.drberkson.com

RESOURCES:

For an appointment with Dr. Burt Berkson, the top expert in the use of alpha lipoic acid for diabetic neuropathy:
Website: www.drberkson.com
Phone: (575) 524-3720

For a high-quality, pharmaceutical-grade ALA (and other) supplements:
Biotech Pharmacal
Website: www.biotechpharmacal.com
Phone: 800-345-1199

Metabolic Maintenance
Website: www.metabolicmaintenance.com
Phone: 800-772-7873

REFERENCES:

1. Golbidi S, et al. Diabetes and alpha lipoic acid. *Frontiers in Pharmacology*, November 2011, Volume 2, Article 69.

2. Gerritje S, et al. Alpha Lipoic Acid for Symptomatic Peripheral Neuropathy in Patients with Diabetes: A Meta-Analysis of Randomized Controlled Trials.

Chapter 15

Coenzyme Q10

New energy for your ailing cells

As we discussed in Chapter 2, there are many factors that can cause diabetes, like being overweight, a sugary diet, nutritional deficiencies and lack of exercise. But more and more experts are saying the cause <u>underlying</u> all those other causes is a problem with your *mitochondria*—and that the best remedy for ailing mitochondria is taking a supplement of *coenzyme Q10.*

What are mitochondria? What is coenzyme Q10? And how can one nutritional supplement fix such a big problem?

Well, if you want to prevent, control or reverse diabetes (and its complications), it's time to find out…

Mitochondria: The powerhouse of the cell

Inside your body are *organs*, each with a specific function. Likewise, inside your cells are *organelles*, super-tiny structures with jobs to do.

The mitochondria—anywhere from 200 to 5,000 per cell—are organelles. And their important job is to *generate energy*—90% of the energy a cell requires.

Most of that energy comes from a compound called adenosine triphosphate, or ATP. ATP is manufactured in a complex, five-step process—a microscopic assembly line of protons and electrons—and that process requires coenzyme Q10 just about every step of the way.

Where does diabetes fit into this picture?

"Since most cellular functions are dependent on an adequate supply of ATP, coenzyme Q10 is essential for the health of virtually all human tissues and organs," wrote Alan Gaby, MD, in his scientific paper *The Role of Coenzyme Q10 in Clinical Medicine.* [1]

And one of those organs is your insulin-producing pancreas.

Your burnt-out beta-cells

Yes, every cell in the body depends on the energy-generating power of mitochondria, including the insulin-producing beta-cells of the pancreas. And if you're among the more than 100 million Americans with prediabetes or diabetes, your beta-cells are probably *tired*.

They no longer produce all the insulin you need *because* they don't have enough ATP… and they don't have enough ATP because the mitochondria inside those cells are falling down on the job…and the mitochondria are underperforming *because* (you guessed it) they don't have enough coenzyme Q10.

But *why* don't they have enough coQ10?

"The body's manufacture of CoQ10 is a complex process, and it requires multiple vitamins, cofactors and amino acids," I was told by Stephen Sinatra, MD, an integrative cardiologist and author of *The Coenzyme Q10 Phenomenon* (and many other books on health and healing). "For example, if the body is deficient in folate, vitamin C, B12 or B6—to name just a few nutrients—the production of coenzyme Q10 could be blocked. Chronic disease can also result in deficiencies. As can environmental stressors. As can taking a cholesterol-lowering statin drug." (You'll read more about statin drugs and what they do to coenzyme Q10 later in this chapter.)

In other words, 21st century life—with its nutrient-poor diets, pollution, diseases and dubious prescription drugs—causes a coenzyme Q10 deficiency.

But if you replenish your body with CoQ10 (as it's popularly called), you'll go a long way toward solving the problem of diabetes. That's because CoQ10 does a lot more than help balance blood sugar.

It also helps supply the energy for the efficient metabolism of carbohydrates, key to blood sugar control.

And it's a powerful antioxidant, protecting cells throughout the body from oxidation, the internal rust that corrodes cells. Oxidation (and inflammation, its evil twin) are rife in diabetes—and they can lead to arterial disease (diabetic arthropathy)…a weakened heart (diabetic cardiomyopathy)…nerve damage (diabetic neuropathy)…kidney disease (diabetic nephropathy)…and eye problems (diabetic retinopathy). CoQ10 can help prevent or even reverse all those health disasters.

But don't take my word for it. Let's review the scientific evidence for the diabetes-beating power of CoQ10…

Defeating diabetes (and its complications) with CoQ10

Better blood sugar control—with 200 mg of daily CoQ10. In a study of nine people with diabetes, four months of daily treatment with 200 milligrams (mg) of CoQ10 lowered A1C from 7.1 to 6.8, a significant drop. (The researchers also gave CoQ10 to five healthy folks—and their ability to produce and use insulin improved.) [2]

In a similar study from Australian researchers, 200 mg of daily CoQ10 significantly lowered A1C. CoQ10 supplementation may improve long-term blood sugar control in people with type 2 diabetes, concluded the researchers in the *European Journal of Clinical Nutrition*. [3]

Nerve pain—prevented. Peripheral neuropathy—sharp, jabbing pain, burning and numbness in the feet and hands—is the most common complication of diabetes. In a study by researchers from the University of Miami School of Medicine, adding CoQ10 to the diets of diabetic rats *completely prevented* diabetic neuropathy. "CoQ10 administration may represent a low-risk, high-reward strategy for preventing or treating diabetic neuropathy," concluded the researchers. [4]

Nerve pain—reversed. In a similar study, 6 months of daily CoQ10 intake *completely reversed* nerve pain in diabetic rats. "Early long-term administration of the antioxidant CoQ10 may represent a promising therapeutic strategy for type 2 diabetes neuropathy," wrote the researchers in the *Proceedings of the National Academy of Sciences*. [5]

Lowering high blood pressure. High blood pressure is common in diabetes, and raises the risk of heart attack and stroke. In a study by Australian researchers, the drug fenofibrate failed to lower blood pressure in diabetes patients. But when the drug was combined with 200 mg of daily CoQ10, blood pressure dropped up to six points. [6]

Another study by the same team of researchers—an analysis of all the studies on CoQ10 and blood pressure—showed the supplement lowers systolic blood pressure by up to 17 points and diastolic pressure by up to 10 points, very sizable decreases. [7]

Reviving sluggish arteries. The *endothelium*—the lining of the arteries—manufactures *nitric oxide*, which relaxes and expands arteries, lowering blood pressure and decreasing the risk of heart attack and stroke. When 40 diabetes patients took 200 mg of CoQ10 for three months, their "endothelial dysfunction" improved and their arterial blood flow increased by nearly 2%, reported Australian doctors. [8]

CoQ10 works to restore the health of the endothelium in diabetes patients because it restores normal function to the mitochondria in endothelial cells and because it's a powerful antioxidant, I was told by Gerald F. Watts, MD, PhD, head of the Department of Internal Medicine and Director of the Lipid Disorders Clinic at Royal Perth Hospital in Australia.

Strengthening a weakened heart. One possible complication of diabetes is *diabetic cardiomyopathy*: Damage to the muscle tissue of the heart, leading to the weak heartbeat of *chronic heart failure*—and almost inevitably to hospitalization and death. In a study from Australian researchers, adding CoQ10 to the diet of diabetic mice strengthened the heartbeat… reduced swollen heart cells…and limited the development of scar tissue in the muscle tissue of the heart. The researchers endorsed "...the addition of coenzyme Q10 to the current therapy used in diabetic patients." [9]

Researchers from Slovakia put that advice into practice, giving 120 mg of daily CoQ10 for three months to 20 people with diabetes —and noted that it strengthened the heart's ability to pump blood. [10]

Protecting the kidneys. Nearly half of people with diabetes develop chronic kidney disease (diabetic nephropathy). In a study by Swedish researchers, supplementing the diet of diabetic rats with CoQ10 "prevented or reduced" mitochondrial damage in the kidneys—and eliminated many of the biomarkers of kidney disease, like poor filtration and excess protein in the urine. These findings highlight "the role of mitochondria" in the development of diabetic kidney disease," wrote the researchers in *Diabetologia*. [11]

And Australian researchers, conducting a similar study, concluded that CoQ10 supplementation may protect the kidneys in type 2 diabetes by preserving mitochondrial function. [12]

CoQ10 deficiency—common in diabetes. Researchers studied 28 diabetes patients and 10 healthy people, and found CoQ10 levels were much lower in those with diabetes—and the lower the level of CoQ10, the higher the level of blood sugar. [13]

Bottom line: If have prediabetes or diabetes, you need CoQ10. Here's how to get it.

The Energy Doctor who relies on CoQ10

Edward Conley, DO, is an assistant clinical professor of medicine at Michigan State University, and medical director of the Fatigue, Fibromyalgia and Autoimmune Clinic in Flint, Michigan, one of the largest chronic fatigue and fibromyalgia clinics in the U.S. He's been prescribing coenzyme Q10 for more than 20 years.

"I started off as a sports medicine physician in 1987 at the U.S. Olympic Training Camp in Lake Placid, helping Olympians increase their energy levels for better performance," he told me. "I soon became very interested in learning how to improve energy levels in *everyone*. That led me to work with people with chronic fatigue syndrome and fibromyalgia—and using CoQ10 to reverse mitochondrial dysfunction and improve energy in those patients."

Dr. Conley explained why a lack of CoQ10 is a perfect setup for getting diabetes. "When you don't have enough CoQ10, you start to feel fatigued—maybe you don't even have enough energy to exercise. Your body also doesn't have enough energy to burn food efficiently, and you start storing it as fat, gaining weight. A sedentary lifestyle and being overweight creates insulin resistance. In this state of prediabetes, your body pumps out more and more insulin until your pancreas exhausts itself—and then you end up with type 2 diabetes.

"And along the way—because you're not burning fats—you probably end up with high cholesterol and are prescribed a cholesterol-lowering statin drug, like Zocor, Lipitor or Mevacor."

Why is that a problem? Because statins *obliterate* CoQ10…

Statins: the drugs that snuff CoQ10

"CoQ10 is made in our bodies along the same pathway as cholesterol," Dr. Conley explained. "So when you take a statin, you not only block the production of cholesterol, you also block the production of CoQ10—which causes even *more* fatigue, *more* trouble burning food for energy, and *more* weight gain." (Not to mention the common side effects of statins like muscle pain and memory loss, directly caused by too little CoQ10 in muscle and brain cells.)

"In Canada, there's a black box warning on statin labels about CoQ10 deficiency, and Canadian doctors *must* prescribe CoQ10 when they prescribe a statin," Dr. Conley continued. "Why Canadians need CoQ10 if they're on statins but Americans don't is a mystery to me. Last I heard, Canadians have the same physiology as Americans.

"Of the tens of millions of Americans with prediabetes and type 2 diabetes, half to three-quarters of them are going to have elevated cholesterol, and most of those people are going to be on statins—and *all* of them could benefit from taking CoQ10."

Controlling the many complications of diabetes

But whether you're on statins or not, deciding to take CoQ10 is a "no-brainer" if you have diabetes, said Dr. Conley.

"CoQ10 is an important nutrient for people who have diabetes but don't have complications. But it's crucial—perhaps even life-saving—for diabetes patients with complications.

"Diabetic complications—to the blood vessels, to the heart, to the nerves, to the kidneys—usually start as an injury to the mitochondria, and CoQ10 can help prevent that.

"I'm all about trying to keep my patients with diabetes from getting the big side effects—

like peripheral neuropathy, cardiomyopathy or kidney disease—by preventing or repairing the damage to mitochondria, and by improving antioxidant status to protect cells.

"The more your readers with diabetes work to prevent mitochondrial and cellular damage from the disease—and taking CoQ10 is a key factor in that prevention—the better the quality of their lives will be over the next 10, 20, 30 or even 40 years.

"And if they already have some damage, they can reverse a lot of it. For example, I've had a number of patients with diabetic neuropathy who have been helped by CoQ10.

"I also put my patients with diabetic cardiomyopathy on high doses of CoQ10, because we're talking about a condition that could be life-ending. To me, that's a very positive therapeutic option, as compared to medicines with toxic side effects or putting the patient in the hospital.

"Information about CoQ10 is *crucial* for everyone with diabetes who is reading your book."

The right dose of the best product

"I typically start my patients with diabetes on 100 milligrams a day of CoQ10, in combination with a better diet and an exercise program," Dr. Conley told me. "Then I look for a response. Does my patient feel any improvement? If they feel more energy and well-being, I increase the amount to 200 to 300 milligrams daily."

But don't rush out and buy yourself some CoQ10—because the product you're buying might be worthless!

"There are hundreds of CoQ10 products out there, and your reader has no way of knowing the quality of those products—and, honestly, neither do I, and neither does anybody else!" Dr. Conley said.

"For example, if I'm a supplement manufacturer, I can go to the Far East, where a lot of CoQ10 is produced, and buy a batch of questionable potency and purity, and put it in a capsule here in the U.S., and sell it—and there's no way to know if it's fabulous or lousy!"

Dr. Conley has solved this problem for his patients: He sells CoQMelt from Douglass labs, which meets all of his specifications for purity and potency.

"This CoQ10 is from Italy, where the quality is consistently good, compared to CoQ10 from the Far East," he said. "It's also the *ubiquinol* form—the type your body makes—which is better absorbed than the *ubiquinone* form.

"I also stock a chewable variety, because my patients seem to like that best. They're taking so many other supplements—this one they can just chew while leaving for work in the morning.

You can order CoQMelt at Dr. Conley's website, www.vitalhealthcenter.com or by phone. (See the Resources section at the end of the chapter for more information.) It is also widely available on the internet.

And don't worry about side effects.

"If you use a decent quality CoQ10, there are no serious side effects, other than a slight lightening of your wallet," said Dr. Conley. "I have prescribed CoQ10 for more than 20 years, and I have never seen a single side effect in my patients, or read any scientific literature documenting side effects."

Plenty of people with diabetes endorse CoQ10

Join the conversation on the internet about CoQ10 for diabetes, and you'll see the supplement typically earns five stars…

Helps neuropathy. "I have been taking 200 mg of CoQ10 daily for diabetes—and it helps my neuropathy a lot," wrote Sherry A.

Pain improved in two days. "My husband has diabetes and has been on statins for cholesterol for five years," wrote Betty M. "A year ago, the aches and pains were so severe that he struggled to even get out of bed. He didn't want to go to a doctor so in desperation I spoke to a local pharmacist who recommended CoQ10. In two days the pain was improved and he could function a lot better."

Can't afford NOT to take it. "As a diabetic, I take CoQ10 for heart health—it's a little bit expensive, but I know I can't afford to shortchange my heart.," wrote Rhonda G.

Works for her and her husband. "CoQ10 is one of the best things for improving circulation," wrote Trudy T. "I was already taking it but not in a big enough dose—I started taking 100 milligrams a day, and it's made a big difference. My husband has diabetic neuropathy and it helps him, too."

Muscle pain from statins—gone. "I was diagnosed with diabetes in 2002 and have been on statin drugs for years," wrote Liz S. I take CoQ10, and it's alleviated all the muscle pain from the statins. It's over-the-counter and a little pricey, but well worth it."

Sleeps better with CoQ10. "I have had diabetes for 29 years and have found that CoQ10 has helped me feel better and actually sleep better," wrote Faye B.

Anti-diabetes secrets in the next chapter...

• Learn how cinnamon is "Mother Nature's herbal insulin"—duplicating the glucose-controlling action of the hormone.

• The most-studied, most effective cinnamon supplement—and the best therapeutic dose.

• How to use the spice for maximum blood glucose control—including dozens of delicious ways to get more cinnamon in your diet.

EXPERTS AND CONTRIBUTORS:

Edward Conley, DO, is an assistant clinical professor of medicine at Michigan State University, medical director of the Fatigue, Fibromyalgia and Autoimmune Clinic in Flint, Michigan, one of the largest chronic fatigue and fibromyalgia clinics in the U.S. He is the author of many self-help health books. His most recent book is *Life Changers: 10 Painless, High-Tech, Home Medical Tests That Can Change Your Life.*
Websites:
www.10lifechangers.com
www.vitalhealthcenter.com
Phone: 810-230-8677
Email: conley@cfids.com

Stephen Sinatra, MD, is an integrative cardiologist and author of *The Coenzyme Q10 Phenomenon* and many other books on health and healing.
Website: www.drsinatra.com

Gerald F. Watts, MD, PhD, is head of the Department of Internal Medicine and Director of the Lipid Disorders Clinic at Royal Perth Hospital in Australia and Winthrop Professor in the Department of Medicine and Pharmacology at the University of Western Australia in Perth.

RESOURCES:

To order high-quality, highly absorbable CoQ10 from Dr. Conley:
Website: www.vitalhealthcenter.com
Phone: (888) 244-3774

REFERENCES:

1. Gaby, AR. The Role of Coenzyme Q10 in Clinical Medicine, Part I. *Alternative Medicine Review*, Volume 1, Number 1, 1996, pages 11-17.

2. Mezawa M, et al. The reduced form of coenzyme Q10 improves glycemic control in patients with type 2 diabetes: an open label pilot study. *Biofactors*, 2012 Nov-Ddec;38(6):416-21.

155

3. Hodgson JM, et al. Coenzyme Q10 improves blood pressure and glycaemic control: a controlled trial in subjects with type 2 diabetes. *European Journal of Clinical Nutrition*, 2002 Nov;56(11):1137-42.

4. Zhang YP, et al. Prophylactic and Antinociceptive Effects of Coenzyme Q10 on Diabetic Neuropathic Pain in a Mouse Model of Type 1 Diabetes. *Anesthesiology*, 2013 Jan 17. [Epub ahead of print]

5. Shi TJ, et al. Coenzyme Q10 prevents peripheral neuropathy and attenuates neuron loss in the db-/db- mouse, a type 2 diabetes model. *Proceedings of the National Academy of Sciences*, 2013 Jan 8;110(2):690-5.

6. Chew GT, et al. Hemodynamic effects of fenofibrate and coenzyme Q10 in type 2 diabetic subjects with left ventricular diastolic dysfunction. *Diabetes Care*, 2008 Aug;31(8):1502-9.

7. Rosenfeld FL, et al. Coenzyme Q10 in the treatment of hypertension: a meta-analysis. *Journal of Human Hypertension*, 2077 Apr;21(4):297-306.

8. Watts GF, et al. Coenzyme Q(10) improves endothelial dysfunction of the brachial artery in Type II diabetes mellitus. *Diabetologia*, 2002 Mar;45(3):420-6.

9. Huynh K, et al. Coenzyme Q10 attenuates diastolic dysfunction, cardiomyocyte hypertrophy and cardiac fibrosis in the db/db mouse model of type 2 diabetes. *Diabetologia,* 2012 May;55(5):1544-53.

10. Palacka P, et al. Complementary therapy in diabetic patients with chronic complications: a pilot study. *Bratisl Lek Listy*, 2010;111(4):205-11.

11. Persson MF, et al. Coenzyme Q10 prevent GDP-sensitive mitochondrial uncoupling, glomerular hyperfiltration and proteinuria in kidneys in db/db mice as a model of type 2 diabetes. *Diabetologia*, 2012 May;55(5):1535-43.

12. Sourris KC, et al. Ubiquinone (coenzyme Q10) prevent renal mitochondrial dysfunction in an experimental model of type 2 diabetes. *Free Radical Biology & Medicine*, 2012 Feb 1;52(3):716-23.

13. El-ghoroury EA, et al. Malondialdehyde and coenzyme Q10 in platelets and serum in type 2 diabetes mellitus: correlation with glycemic control. *Blood Coagulation & Fibrinolysis*, 2009 Jun;20(4):248-51.

PART IV

Herbal Diabetes Cures

Move over pharmaceuticals.
Mother Nature makes the most powerful
anti-diabetes medicines.

Chapter 16

Cinnamon

To balance your blood sugar, just add spice.

The last time I wrote about cinnamon and diabetes was for my book *Breakthroughs in Natural Healing 2012*, and I interviewed my favorite expert on the topic: Richard Anderson, PhD, CNS, a Lead Scientist at the USDA's Beltsville Human Nutrition Research Center in Maryland. He's the author of 29 scientific papers (and counting) on the use of cinnamon to prevent and control blood sugar problems.

Needless to say, Dr. Anderson knows something about the glucose-regulating power of cinnamon, a spice derived from the bark of a tropical evergreen tree. So I called him again while writing this Special Report, and asked him to update me on the how and the why of this amazing spice.

"Cinnamon *mimics* the action of insulin, the hormone that controls blood sugar," he reminded me. "It stimulates insulin receptors on cells the same way insulin does, allowing excess sugar to move out of the blood and into cells."

In 2010, Dr. Anderson and a few of his colleagues summarized all the research to date on cinnamon and diabetes, in a paper titled "Cinnamon: potential role in the prevention of insulin resistance, metabolic syndrome and type 2 diabetes," published in the *Journal of Diabetes Science and Technology*. [1]

The evidence they assembled shows that cinnamon can…

Improve long-term blood sugar levels in type 2 diabetes. In a three-month study of more than 100 diabetes patients, cinnamon lowered A1C by 0.83%—a decrease that lowers the risk of heart disease by 16%, eye problems (diabetic retinopathy) by 20% and kidney disease (diabetic nephropathy) by 30%. Not a bad day's work for a spice you can find in any kitchen!

Improve metabolic syndrome. In a three-month study of people with the metabolic syndrome, cinnamon lowered average blood sugar levels by 10 points—10 times more than people taking a placebo, who had virtually no change. After three months, the folks taking cinnamon also had lower blood pressure and less body fat.

Decrease spikes in glucose levels after eating. High, post-meal levels of blood sugar are a sign of advancing diabetes and—because they damage arteries—a risk factor for heart disease. In one study, adding cinnamon to a meal of rice pudding cut the post-meal spike in blood sugar by nearly 30 points, compared to a meal without cinnamon.

Improve risk factors for heart disease. Studies show that adding cinnamon to the diet lowers total cholesterol; lowers bad LDL cholesterol; increases good HDL cholesterol; lowers triglycerides; and lowers high blood pressure.

Dr. Anderson's scientific conclusion: "Cinnamon may be important in the prevention and alleviation of the signs and symptoms of metabolic syndrome, type 2 diabetes and cardiovascular and related diseases."

About a year after Dr. Anderson's paper appeared, researchers from the Department of Nutrition at the University of California, Davis, analyzed eight studies on the use of cinnamon in prediabetes and diabetes. [2] Their conclusion echoed Dr. Anderson's:

"Cinnamon extract and/or cinnamon improves fasting blood glucose in people with prediabetes or type 2 diabetes."

The most powerful form of cinnamon

Of the 11 studies on people reviewed by Dr. Anderson, five of them tested a unique cinnamon extract—a *water* extract of the spice, called *Cinsulin*.

"Cinsulin is 20 times more powerful at sparking insulin activity than any other tested herb, spice or medicinal extract," Dr. Anderson told me.

What's the secret behind Cinsulin?

The insulin-activating parts of cinnamon—*catechin, epicatechin* and *procyanidin* and other plant compounds collectively known as *polyphenols*—are found mostly in the watery part of the spice, not in the oil, Dr. Anderson explained. The water extract concentrates these compounds, giving cinnamon added glucose-controlling power.

Dr. Anderson's research on animals shows that the water extract works in a couple of different ways. It…

- Improves insulin signaling—the ability of insulin receptors on the outside of cells to communicate with the hormone.

- Boosts nitric oxide, a glucose-regulating compound.

- Regulates genes involved in blood sugar control.

- Blocks immune factors that play a role in insulin resistance.

The extract is also a powerful antioxidant, protecting cells from damaging oxidation and inflammation, which play a role not only in diabetes, but also in heart disease, cancer and Alzheimer's disease. (Laboratory research shows the water extract can protect animals from those diseases.)

In one of the largest studies on Cinsulin, researchers at Oklahoma State University gave 137 diabetes patients a daily dose of either 500 milligrams (mg) of Cinsulin or a placebo. After two months, the Cinsulin group had a 7.5% drop in fasting blood sugar, compared with a 1.6% drop in the placebo group. Cinsulin also controlled post-meal glucose spikes. [3]

This study "adds to the growing evidence that aqueous [water] cinnamon extract may be beneficial for insulin-resistant populations," said Barbara Stoecker, PhD, a study researcher.

How much Cinsulin do you need? Most studies use 500 mg a day. Take one 250 mg capsule with breakfast and one with lunch or dinner, advises Dr. Anderson.

Cinsulin is widely available on the internet and in retail stores like Costco and GNC.

Adding cinnamon to your diet

But you don't need to buy a special supplement to reap the benefits of cinnamon. You can just use the spice itself—either in a capsule or with food.

"Try to get ¼ to 1 teaspoon of cinnamon daily, the amount used in most studies," Dr. Anderson said. "Sprinkle it in hot cereals, yogurt or applesauce. Use it to accent sweet potatoes, winter squash or yams. Try it with lamb, beef stew or chilies. It even goes great with grains such as couscous and barley, and legumes such as lentils and split peas."

You can buy cinnamon either as sticks (harvested, dried bark that has been rolled into *quills*) or cinnamon powder (ground quills).

"If you buy quills, look for ones that are tightly rolled, evenly colored and blemish free," I was told by Deborah Yost, co-author of *Healing Spices*. "Once ground, cinnamon begins to lose the wonderful fragrance and flavor that comes from its volatile oils, so it's best to buy whole quills and grind them as needed. The quills are somewhat tough, so you'll need a quality spice grinder."

"If you buy ground cinnamon, you'll get the most fragrance and flavor from the finest quality, which is smooth rather than gritty," she continued.

"Whole quills keep for three years, as long as they aren't in extreme heat. Ground cinnamon begins to fade in flavor after a few months."

Yost offered these ideas for eating more cinnamon:

Sprinkle on apples, bananas, melons and oranges. Mix with mint and parsley in ground beef for burgers and meatloaf. Mix into rice pilaf. Put a cinnamon quill in beef or vegetarian stews, or in lentil soup. Combine equal parts cinnamon, cardamom and black pepper and rub into pork tenderloin or lamb before baking. Add to hot cocoa to enhance the flavor of the chocolate. Sprinkle into pastry dough for pies and quiches. Make spiced tea: put a quart of brewed tea in a pot, add two cups of apple juice, a lemon slice and two cinnamon sticks; simmer gently for 10 minutes.

"I've had my insulin intake reduced twice."

That comment is pretty representative of the type of cinnamon-flavored testimonial from diabetes patients that you can find on the internet. A few examples…

No more diabetes medicine. "I put about 2 teaspoons of cinnamon in my coffee filter and then put coffee grounds on top," says a post at www.peoplespharmacy.com. "I get the benefits of the cinnamon and it cuts any bitterness from the coffee. I turned all my family and friends on to this—and my mother-in-law was able to go off the diabetes medicine that she's been on for years!"

A1C down 2%. "My diabetes educator said cinnamon would be good for me," says a post at www.diabeticconnect.com. "I take just 2 capsules a day in the morning—1000 milligrams—along with fish oil. My A1C has dropped 2 points, down to 7.6 percent—and I've lost 10 pounds!"

The doctor was so impressed, she put her husband on cinnamon. "I read about taking cinnamon to help with controlling my diabetes," says another post at www.diabeticconnect.com. "Well, finally I tried it. After about six weeks of taking 1000 mg two times a day—my long-term test was in control! It has been ever since—and I've even had my insulin intake reduced twice! My doctor is very pleased—and even put her diabetic husband on cinnamon."

More cinnamon, less insulin. "My mom uses cinnamon capsules for her diabetes—it does help quite a bit," says a post at www.welltrainedmind.com. "I notice she takes less insulin when she consistently takes the cinnamon."

Check it out! "My husband is diabetic and controls his blood sugar level with cinnamon capsules," says a post at www.healthexpertadvice.org. "Really—cinnamon! Check it out."

Anti-diabetes secrets in the next chapter...

- Ninety percent of hard-to-heal diabetic skin ulcers *completely* healed—with Pycnogenol, a powerful antioxidant from tree bark.

- How to *prevent* foot ulcers with Pycnogenol.

- Six studies, 1,300 people—and proof positive that Pycnogenol can stop the progression of diabetic eye disease. (And improve vision!)

- The remarkable story of the woman with diabetes who could hardly walk—and who is DANCING again after taking Pycnogenol.

EXPERTS AND CONTRIBUTORS:

Richard Anderson, PhD, is a Lead Scientist in the Diet, Genomics, and Immunology Laboratory of the Beltsville Human Nutrition Research Center, a division of the United States Department of Agriculture.

Deborah Yost is the co-author of *Healing Spices* and many other health books.

REFERENCES:

1. Qin B, et al. Cinnamon: potential role in the prevention of insulin resistance, metabolic syndrome, and type 2 diabetes. *Journal of Diabetes Science and Technology,* 2010 May 1;4(3):685-93.

2. Davis PA, et al. Cinnamon intake lowers fasting blood glucose: meta-analysis. *Journal of Medicinal Food,* 2011 Sep;14(9):884-9.

3. Stoecker B, et al. Cinnamon extract lowers blood glucose in hyperglycemic subjects. *Journal of the Federation of American Societies for Experimental Biology (FASEB),* 2010 April; 24 (1): 722.1.

Chapter 17

Pycnogenol

Breakthrough treatment for diabetic foot ulcers—and much more

Like millions of other Americans, I watched the 2012 HBO documentary, "Weight of the Nation," about the obesity crisis. It included many interviews with people plagued by extra pounds, telling their sad tales of disability and disease. One of the saddest was told by Mary and Dan Hanley, a couple in their 60s.

(Viewer discretion advised: Their story, which follows, is grim. But hang on, because I've got a solution for you—you *don't* have to suffer what Mary and Dan did.)

"We were overweight," Mary says, sitting at her dining room table with Dan by her side, looking distraught and sick. "And it just takes a little bit of overweight to start the diabetes, to lose a toe, then to have bypasses in the leg, and trying to save it, and then losing a foot…"

The scene switches to the Hanley's bedroom, with Dan in his wheelchair. We see the stump of his amputated leg…his prosthetic on the floor …and Mary wheeling him into the bathroom and shutting the door behind him. "You learn there are some things you can do and some things you can't," she says.

Next, we accompany Dan on a visit to his doctor—David Nathan, MD, director of the Diabetes Center at Massachusetts General Hospital in Boston. "Diabetes affects the *blood vessels*," Dr. Nathan tells us, "and it affects the vessels supplying the eye, the vessels supplying the kidney, maybe the vessels supplying the nervous system—those are the small vessels. And then it also affects those medium-sized vessels that supply circulation to the heart, to the brain, and to the legs, the *periphery*.

"The peripheral nervous system is what gives you *sensation*," he continues. "So people with diabetes suffer from peripheral neuropathy, which means that they don't feel their toes as well—they don't have the same sensitivity to light touch or to temperature—and their feet are therefore very vulnerable to various kinds of trauma."

Segue back to Mary and Dan, once again sitting at the dining room table. "You don't realize all that can go wrong when you are a diabetic," Mary says. "In 2010, January—actually it was New Year's weekend—and he woke up at about 3:00 in the morning, and his foot had mushroomed to twice its size. We called his primary care doctor and he said, 'Get in immediately, I'll have the vascular team set up.' Which he did, in the emergency room. They took a look at his foot and said, 'If it's between your life and your foot, your foot goes.'"

Once again, we're back in the hospital with Dan and Dr. Nathan, who first examines Dan's stump and then looks at a big skin ulcer on his remaining foot. "There's this risk that we know of," says Dr. Nathan, "that about 50 percent of people with an amputation on the one side will get an amputation on the other side within about five years or so..."

Four million foot ulcers

Like I said, it's a sad story. But maybe even sadder is the fact that it's also the story of *millions* of other people with diabetes. Consider these shocking statistics…

About 15% of people with diabetes—that's four million Americans—will develop ulcers on the skin of their feet. And because those ulcers are so difficult to close and heal, they're also the most common cause of hospitalization for people with diabetes.

For many people (like Dan Hanley) they *don't* heal. About 2% of diabetes patients have a foot or leg amputated when a foot ulcer doesn't close, gets larger, gets infected, and the infection becomes life-threatening.

Two percent may not sound like many. But that's 65,000 amputations. *Every year.*

Foot ulcers require a range of self-care and medical care, all of which you should discuss with your doctor.

But there's one healing option your doctor is unlikely to know about or recommend—even though published research shows it may work *better* to heal foot ulcers than standard care. The option:

Pycnogenol, a patented combo of more than *three dozen* antioxidants, extracted from the bark of the French maritime pine tree.

A new option for healing foot ulcers

"Pycnogenol, a potent antioxidant, is one of the most well-researched natural health supplements available," I was told by Frank Schonlau, PhD, scientific director for Horphag Research, the producer of Pycnogenol. He's not exaggerating. There are more than 100 scientific studies on the benefits of Pycnogenol—including two studies on its power to help heal foot ulcers in diabetes.

Complete healing of foot ulcers after six weeks. In one of those studies, doctors from universities in Italy and Germany treated 30 people with diabetic foot ulcers, using four different approaches:

1. Pycnogenol, taken as a supplement and topically applied to the ulcer.

2. Pycnogenol, only taken as supplement.

3. Pycnogenol, only used topically.

4. Standard medications for foot ulcers, like antibiotics.

Of those receiving the combined Pycnogenol treatment, 89% had *complete healing* of their foot ulcers after six weeks. The rate was 85% with the supplement alone, and 84% with topical application alone. But only 61% of those receiving standard medication had total healing.

"Combined systemic and local application of Pycnogenol may offer a new treatment for diabetic ulcers," concluded the researchers. [1]

Pycnogenol works by increasing *microcirculation* (the delivery of blood to the tiniest blood vessels), bringing healing oxygen and nutrients to the ulcer.

"The Pycnogenol groups all showed a significantly increased oxygen presence in the skin," said Dr. Gianni Belcaro, who led the study.

Preventing foot ulcers. The second study provided more proof of Pycnogenol's power to improve microcirculation. The same team of doctors gave either Pycnogenol or a placebo to 60 people with diabetes who didn't have foot ulcers. Those taking the supplement had a greater increase in the microcirculation of their feet; those taking the placebo didn't.

Because it improves microcirculation, Pycnogenol may also help *prevent* diabetic foot ulcers, concluded the researchers. [2]

My advice as a health coach to my clients with diabetes: Pycnogenol is a supplement you should seriously consider taking. And not just for the sake of your feet…

Foot ulcers linked to heart attacks and strokes

Foot ulcers are an obvious sign of circulatory problems, which is why researchers in England studied more than 18,000 people with diabetes to see if the folks with foot ulcers were at greater risk for other disasters of poor circulation, like heart attacks and strokes. Their findings are important to take into account. If you're a diabetes patient with a foot ulcer, you're…

- 222% more likely to die of a heart attack

- 41% more likely to die of a stroke

- 89% more likely to die of any cause

"Our research, which is the largest and therefore most reliable study to date, shows that people with diabetes who have foot ulcers are at considerably higher risk of an earlier death compared to those patients without foot ulcers," said Robert Hinchliffe, MD, at St. George's Vascular Institute in London, who led the study. "We suspect that this may be due in part to the greater co-existence of cardiovascular disease and foot ulcers with diabetes, as well as the effect of infections among those with foot ulcers."

"Our results warrant further investigation as to whether even greater control of risk factors, such as high blood pressure and high blood glucose, can further reduce mortality among those with foot ulcers," added Kausik Ray, MD, another study author.

Well, the good news is that Pycnogenol can help control those risk factors, too.

Helping your heart, lowering your blood sugar

The medical database of the National Institutes of Health features many studies that used Pycnogenol to improve the risk factors of heart disease and lower blood sugar levels…

Healthier hearts in diabetes—and lower blood sugar, too. Researchers at the University of Arizona gave 48 diabetes patients with high blood pressure either 125 mg of Pycnogenol or a placebo. After three months, 58% of those taking the supplement had normal blood pressure. (And those still on blood pressure medication could take less of it.)

Additionally, A1C (a measure of long-term blood sugar control) dropped *eight times more* in the Pycnogenol group. Fasting glucose dropped *four times more* among those taking Pycnogenol—with an average drop of 23.7. Bad LDL cholesterol dropped by 13.

"Pycnogenol," concluded the researchers, "resulted in lowered cardiovascular risk factors, improved diabetes control and reduced antihypertensive [blood pressure] medicine." [4]

Better circulation in people with heart disease. Twenty-three people with heart disease who took 200 milligrams (mg) a day of Pycnogenol for two months had a 25% improvement in the ability of arteries to relax and expand, improving blood flow. They also had an 8% drop in a biomarker of oxidation (free radical damage). [5]

Stopping vision loss in diabetes. Although the focus of this chapter is foot ulcers, problems with microcirculation can also affect the eyes, as Dr. Nathan pointed out. The condition is called *diabetic retinopathy*—damage to the tiny blood vessels in the retina, the back part of the eye that changes light into nerve signals. It affects 40 to 45% of people with diabetes, and it's a leading cause of vision problems—including blindness.

You can shield your eyes with Pycnogenol.

There have been six studies on diabetic retinopathy and Pycnogenol, involving nearly 1,300 people with diabetes. "All of these studies showed that Pycnogenol can stop the progression of retinopathy and improve vision," Dr. Schonlau told me. It works by strengthening weakened blood vessels and reducing leaking into the retina—the cause of the vision problems. In fact, Pycnogenol worked just as well as a drug commonly used for the disease.

In the most recent study, 24 people with diabetic retinopathy took Pycnogenol for three months. They had significant improvements in three measurements of the severity of the problem—less accumulation of fluid in the retina; less thickness of the retina; and better blood flow in the retinal artery. They also had better vision: 18 of the 24 patients said they could see better; and measurements on an eye chart improved by 18%.

"Pycnogenol taken at the early stage of retinopathy may enhance retinal blood circulation, accompanied by regression of edema [fluid accumulation], which favorably improves vision of patients," wrote the study researchers. [6]

Lowering blood sugar in prediabetes. Italian doctors studied 64 people with metabolic syndrome, giving them 150 mg of Pycnogenol daily; another 66 people with metabolic syndrome didn't take the supplement. [7] After six months…

• Blood sugar levels dropped from 123 to 106.

• Waist sizes slimmed by 8%

• Triglycerides and blood pressure fell, and HDL increased.

• Free radicals—cell-damaging molecules—fell by 35%.

"This extraordinary supplement can prevent or reduce the risk of chronic disease triggered by free radicals," I was told by Steven Lamm, MD, a practicing internist, faculty member at the New York University School of Medicine, and Director of Men's Health for the NYU Medical Center.

"What I have come to like so much about Pycnogenol is its broad spectrum of health benefits," he continued. "In addition to its powerful antioxidant effects—which help in protecting against diabetes, heart disease, cancer and other diseases linked to the chemical action of free radicals—it also strengthens tiny capillaries, the blood vessels that help nourish cells, thereby addressing many of the complications of diabetes, like peripheral neuropathy and foot ulcers."

"After six months her neuropathy had vanished—and she could dance again."

Dr. Lamm isn't the only doctor who is excited by Pycnogenol. Another physician who raves about the supplement is Fred Pescatore, MD, who practices nutritional medicine in New York City, and is the author of the bestselling *Hamptons Diet* and many other books.

"Diabetes causes *microangiopathy*—the destruction of the smallest blood vessels, or capillaries," Dr. Pescatore told me. "That's why you get peripheral neuropathy and foot ulcers… why the eyes go bad…why men with diabetes get erectile dysfunction. Pycnogenol works on that level of microcirculation—and that's why we see such great results with it in diabetes."

Dr. Pescatore suggests taking 100 to 200 mg of the supplement daily, which is the range used in most of the studies described in this chapter. In severe cases, the higher end of that range may be more effective. (Pycnogenol is available in a wide range of supplements from many different manufacturers.) For example…

"I treated one woman with diabetes who had severe peripheral neuropathy—numbness and tingling in her legs, and postural and walking problems," he told me. "She took 200 milligrams a day, and after about six months she said her neuropathy had *vanished*—she could stand upright and walk. In fact, she could *dance*, which is something she loved to do and had to stop doing because she had become so unsure on her feet and would trip. That was one of my most impressive cases using Pycnogenol to treat diabetes."

"I suffered with severe burning in both feet—and I have no more burning."

There are plenty of other folks with diabetes who have enjoyed similar benefits using Pycnogenol, many of whom are discussing their newfound health on the internet…

No more burning. "I have diabetes and suffered with severe burning in both feet and legs," says a post at www.webmd.com. "I started taking 30 milligrams of Pycnogenol twice a day—and I have no more burning. If I miss taking it for two or three days, the burning pain comes back. I try to always have one extra bottle around so I don't run out."

Leg cramps gone. "I've had diabetes for 15 years," says a post at www.lowcarber.org. "I used to have severe nighttime leg cramps in both legs, due to diabetic microangiopathy. My endocrinologist recommended 30 milligrams of Pycnogenol before bedtime. I've been taking it for 14 months, and I haven't had a cramp since—starting on the very first night!"

Saved my sight. "Diabetes is tough!" says a post at www.diabetes.co.uk. "Have a look at the supplement Pycnogenol. Studies have shown for a long time it has serious benefits for sight issues, as well as being good for health. I read up on it and have taken it daily since I lost the sight in one eye. <u>I believe it has saved my remaining sight</u>.”

Cholesterol down. “I am 67 and take 100 milligrams of Pycnogenol every day,” says a post at <u>www.topix.com</u>. “I got my cholesterol and my diabetes down to normal after eight months. Try it. <u>Pycnogenol is the future</u>.”

Anti-diabetes secrets in the next chapter...

- Discover how the herb fenugreek rivals the sugar-lowering levels of diabetes medicines.

- Is fenugreek just as effective as diet and exercise? One provocative study says so.

- When a drug failed, the drug *and* fenugreek worked, say these doctors.

- Typical response: a 60 to 80 point drop in blood sugar levels, in four months. “Powerful,” says this nutritionist.

EXPERTS AND CONTRIBUTORS:

Robert Hinchliffe, MD, is a senior lecturer and consultant in vascular surgery at St. George’s Vascular Institute in London.

Steven Lamm, MD, is a practicing internist, faculty member at the New York University School of Medicine, and Director of Men’s Health for the NYU Medical Center.
Website: www.drstevenlamm.com

Fred Pescatore, MD, is a traditionally-trained physician who practices nutritional medicine. He is the author of the *New York Times* bestselling book *The Hamptons Diet* and many other books, and the Reality Health Check newsletter.
Website: www.drpescatore.com

Kausik Ray, MD, is professor of Cardiovascular Disease Prevention at St. George’s Hospital in London.

Frank Schonlau, PhD, is the scientific director for Horphag Research, the producer of Pycnogenol, one of the most well-researched natural health supplements.

REFERENCES:

1. Belcaro G, et al. Diabetic ulcers: microcirculatory improvement and faster healing with Pycnogenol. *Clinical and Applied Thrombosis/Hemostasis*, 2006 Jul;12(3):318-23.

2. Cesarone MR, et al. Improvement of diabetic microangiopathy with Pycnogenol: a prospective controlled study.

3. Brownrigg JR, et al. The association of ulceration of the foot with cardiovascular and all-cause mortality in patients with diabetes: a meta-analysis. *Diabetolgoia*, 2012;55 (11):2906.

4. Zibadi S, et al. Reduction of cardiovascular risk factors in subjects with type 2 diabetes by Pycnogenol supplementation. *Nutrition Research*, 2008 May;28(5):315-20.

5. Enseleit F, et al. Effects of Pycnogenol on endothelial function in patients with stable coronary artery disease: a double-blind, randomized, placebo-controlled, cross-over study. *European Heart Journal*, 2012 Jul;33(13):1589-97.

6. Steigerwalt R, et al. Pycnogenol improves microcirculation, retinal edema, and visual acuity in early diabetic retinopathy. *Journal of Ocular Pharmacology and Therapy*, 2009 Dec;25(6):537-40.

7. Belcaro G, et al. Pycnogenol Supplementation Improves Health Risk Factors in Subjects with Metabolic Syndrome. *Phytotherapy Research*, 2013 Jan 28. [Epub ahead of print]

Chapter 18

Fenugreek

An ancient herb with modern medicinal power

Fenugreek is a plant with a planetary pedigree.

The ancient Egyptians used it to embalm mummies. The ancient Romans, on the other hand, used it calm mommies, giving it to women in labor to ease birth. In traditional Chinese medicine, fenugreek is touted as tonic. Ditto for Ayurveda, the ancient system of natural healing from India, a country where they also put fenugreek seeds and leaves to culinary use, in chutneys and curries. And in Ireland they say that fiber-rich fenugreek seeds "exert anti-diabetic effects."

Yes, that's the 21st century scientific take on fenugreek, from researchers at the University of Ulster in Northern Ireland, writing in the *British Journal of Nutrition*. They're just one of many scientific teams from around the world that have conducted studies on fenugreek and diabetes, now numbering in the hundreds. Those studies, on animals and people, show fenugreek can...

- **Fight cell-damaging oxidants.**

- **Increase enzymes that help regulate blood sugar.**

- **Activate insulin signaling in fat cells and liver cells**, a key to blood sugar regulation. "Fenugreek may hold promise" for people with prediabetes, lessening the chance they'll progress to type 2 diabetes, said a report on the herb in *Alternative Medicine Review*. [1]

- **Balance daily blood sugar levels.** "Our results show that the action of fenugreek in lowering blood glucose levels is almost comparable to the effect of insulin," wrote a team of researchers in the *Journal of Biosciences*. [2]

- **Lower long-term blood sugar levels.** A roundup of all the studies on fenugreek, published in the *Journal of Ethnopharmacology,* showed that it can lower long-term blood sugar levels (A1C) by 1.13%—rivaling the power of many diabetes medicines. [3]

- **Slow diabetic retinopathy**, eye damage that can lead to poor vision and blindness.

Fenugreek also lowers risk factors for heart disease, the #1 killer of people with diabetes. Research shows fenugreek can…

- Lower total cholesterol.

- Lower bad LDL cholesterol

- Lower VLDL, a particularly nasty type of LDL.

- Increase good HDL cholesterol.

- Lower triglycerides, another heart-hurting blood fat.

- Thin blood, reducing the risk of blood clots.

Fenugreek—better than diet and exercise?

In one standout study, doctors at India's Jaipur Diabetes Center divided 25 people newly diagnosed with diabetes into two groups. One group received a daily 1,000 milligram (mg) dose of fenugreek seed extract; the other group started a diet and exercise program. Two months later, both groups had substantial drops in daily glucose levels (the fenugreek group went from 148 to 119).

But the fenugreek group had much better insulin numbers—56% lower levels of insulin… 19% less insulin resistance…and 19% more insulin sensitivity. [4]

Although it's far from conclusive proof, the study "suggests that fenugreek seeds and diet/exercise may be equally effective strategies for attaining glycemic control," said a report on the study from Natural Standard, which provides information about complementary and alternative medicine.

"Remarkable" results that a drug couldn't achieve

In another demonstration of fenugreek's glucose-taming talents, Chinese doctors studied 69 diabetes patients whose disease wasn't well-controlled with sulfonylurea drugs. They divided the patients into two groups: 46 took the drug *and* a fenugreek extract; 23 took the drug and a placebo. [5]

After three months, those taking fenugreek, had "remarkable decreases" in fasting blood glucose…post-meal glucose levels…A1C…and diabetes symptoms, said the researchers.

"The combined therapy" of a fenugreek extract with an anti-diabetic drug "could lower the blood glucose level and ameliorate clinical symptoms in the treatment of type 2 diabetes," concluded the researchers in the *Chinese Journal of Integrative Medicine*.

"Truly an amazing product."

The two products favored by health professionals I talked with are available only *from* health professionals, which is a good indication of their quality and effectiveness. They are:

- Fen-Gre, from Standard Process.

- Fenugreek Plus, from Metagenics.

"Fenugreek is a powerful regulator of blood sugar and blood fats," I was told by Thomas Von Ohlen, MS, a nutritionist with a private practice in Fairfield, Connecticut and a worldwide consulting service. "And because it's so potent, fenugreek can create significant changes in blood sugar levels in just a few months—even without a lot of other changes in diet or exercise.

"For example, I treated a diabetes patient with fenugreek, and with several other natural modalities that strengthened his liver and adrenal glands. His blood glucose went from the high 100s to 95 in two months—a *very* significant drop.

"And that's not an unusual result in my experience with fenugreek," he continued. "The typical response is a 60 to 80 point drop in fasting blood sugar levels within four months—a *huge* drop.

"I like to use the Fenugreek product from Standard Process, because the company has been around for 80 years, they grow the materials for their plant-based supplements on a 1,000-acre organic farm, and they're very thorough in checking every batch for purity."

Ohlen recommends taking three capsules before breakfast, before lunch and before dinner, with the approval and supervision of a health professional. And he recommends *always* taking a fenugreek supplement with 12 ounces of water. "That helps it get into the system and start working a lot faster," he said.

"This is truly an amazing product—one of the 'miracle' products out there," he continued. "Seeing such a big drop in blood sugar levels in just a few months, for a chronic health problem like diabetes, is pretty remarkable."

He also recommends fenugreek for anyone with prediabetes. "By taking fenugreek when you're in a prediabetic situation, you have a much better chance of regulating your blood sugar over time."

Brad Davison, vice-president of Metabolism and Performance Research at Stark Training in Irvine, California, uses fenugreek with clients to help keep blood sugar and insulin balanced. "I like to use Fenugreek Plus, from Metagenics, because I've found it to work really well in balancing blood sugar," he told me. "It combines fenugreek and other herbs that aid in insulin sensitivity." He recommends 2 capsules, three times a day, with meals.

(To find health professionals who use Standard Process and Metagenics products, please see the "Resources" section at the end of the chapter.)

Fans of fenugreek

You can find a lot of fans of fenugreek on the web—or relatives of fans...

Starting the day with fenugreek. "My mom and aunt controlled their sugar levels with medicines, dietary changes and fenugreek," says a post at www.healthexpertadvice.org. "Every morning, they drink warm, fenugreek seed water—they boil two teaspoons of fenugreek seeds in a big glass of water at night and drink it the next morning. Now they're at the point where they don't need medicine—they just control the sugars with diet and fenugreek."

Lowered A1C 3%—and helped with Parkinson's, too. "I started taking 1 teaspoon of roasted fenugreek seeds three times a day, before meals," says a post at www.dailystrength. org. "Plus, I also soak 1 teaspoon of fenugreek seeds in a cup of water at night and drink the water first thing in the morning. My diabetes level has dropped from 10.9 to 7.9. And I feel some improvement in my Parkinson's."

His mentor recommends it. "My diabetes mentor is type 1," says another post at the site. "He recommends fenugreek—both as a supplement and a vegetable—and says it lowers blood sugar as well as the metformin."

Husband and wife both like fenugreek (for very different reasons). "My DH [dear husband] is diabetic and he drinks fenugreek tea, which is good for sugar level control," says a post at www.longhaircommunity.com. "I boil the fenugreek powder and water for a few minutes, let it sit for half an hour, and then he drinks the tea. I save the powder and some water for my hair, and let it sit for a few hours, until it becomes kind of mucous. Then I apply it on my hair and leave it for about 20 minutes, then rinse well. It leaves my hair soft and smooth and I love it."

A remedy they want to share. "The best way to take diabetes in control is exercise and diet," says a post from a new member at www.diabetesdaily.com. "Apart from that, there are a few things that have benefitted us in controlling diabetes, which we want to share with u all. And one of them is fenugreek seeds—half a tablespoon, soaked in water overnight, and drink the water every morning." (The writer's other recommendations include cinnamon, oats for breakfast, and half an avocado before bedtime.)

Anti-diabetes secrets in the next chapter...

- Blood sugar levels drop 15% in two hours—with the herb banaba.

- Amazing long-term results from multiple studies: 30% drop in blood sugar after two weeks…prediabetes reversed…a one-year study showing long-lasting effects…and more.

- The most effective dose of corosolic acid (the active ingredient in banaba) for controlling blood sugar—and how to make sure your supplement delivers it.

EXPERTS AND CONTRIBUTORS:

Brad Davison is vice-president of Metabolism and Performance Research at Stark Training in Irvine, California.
Website: www.starktraining.com

Thomas Von Ohlen, MS, is a nutritionist with a private practice in Fairfield, Connecticut and a worldwide, web-phone based nutritional consulting service.
Website: www.healyourbodynow.com

RESOURCES:

To find a health professional who uses Standard Process products with clients and patients:
Website: www.standardprocess.com

To find a health professional who uses Metagenics Products with clients and patients:
Website: www.metagenics.com

REFERENCES:

1. Basch E, et al. Therapeutic applications of fenugreek. *Alternative Medicine Review*, 2003, Vol. 8, #1.

2. Baquer NZ, et al. Metabolic and molecular action of Trigonella foenum-graecum (fenugreek) and trace metals in experimental diabetic tissues. *Journal of Biosciences*, 2011 Jun;36(2):383-96.

3. Suksomboon N, et al. Meta-analysis of the effect of herbal supplement on glycemic control in type 2 diabetes. *Journal of Ethnopharmacology*, 2011 Oct 11;137(3):1328-33.

4. Gupta A, et al. Effect of Trigonella foenum-graccum (fenugreek) seeds on glycaemic control and insulin resistance in type 2 diabetes mellitus: a double blind placebo controlled study. *Journal of the Association of Physicians of India*, 2001 Nov;49:1057-61.

5. Lu FR, et al. Clinical observation on trigonella foenum-graecum L. total saponins in combination with sulfonylureas in the treatment of type 2 diabetes. *Chinese Journal of Integrative Medicine*, 2008 Mar;14(1):56-60.

Chapter 19

Banaba

A folk remedy for the 21ˢᵗ century

Dr. Sid Stohs knows something about nutritional and herbal supplements.

Dean Emeritus of Creighton University Medical Center in Omaha, Nebraska, Dr. Stohs has a master's degree in pharmacognosy (the study of natural products as medicines), a PhD in biochemistry, and is also an expert in nutrition, pharmacology and toxicology (the side effects of medicines and other compounds). For five years, he was the senior vice-president for research and development at AdvoCare, a maker of health products, where he formulated 25 new supplements and other natural products and upgraded another 40 or so.

Although he's retired, Dr. Stohs is still very interested in the science of supplements for health and healing, and regularly writes "review" articles for scientific journals that summarize all the current knowledge about a particular nutrient or herb.

His most recent review article, published in 2012, is on *banaba*, a plant from the Philippines with a long history as a folk remedy, with the locals using the leafy bush to make tea for diabetes and other health problems. [1]

(Here in the U.S.—where it's called the Crape Myrtle—it's widely grown as an ornamental, with thick bouquets of red, white, lavender or purple flowers that bloom in the summer and fall.)

So when I wanted to find out if banaba was the real deal, I emailed Dr. Stohs, asking if he'd be willing to talk to me about his findings. He was—and here's what he had to say, both on the phone and in his scientific review.

Banaba: Scientific research shows that it works

"I was amazed by how much research has been done on banaba, both in animals and humans," he told me. Some highlights of the research on people…

A drop in blood sugar—and fewer symptoms of diabetes. Chinese researchers studied 100 people with prediabetes and diabetes, dividing them into two groups. Half took a daily banaba extract standardized for corosolic acid (the active ingredient in banaba) and half took a placebo. After one month, the average fasting and post-meal glucose levels of those taking banaba were 10% lower than the placebo group. They also had fewer symptoms of diabetes, like thirst, fatigue and hunger. [1]

Lower blood sugar in 90 minutes. Thirty-one people (19 with diabetes; 8 with prediabetes; and 4 with no blood sugar problems) were given 10 mg of corosolic acid or a placebo. Ninety minutes later, those taking corosolic acid had much lower blood sugar levels. [2]

30% drop in blood sugar—in two weeks. Researchers in Florida gave 10 people with diabetes either 32 or 48 milligrams (mg) daily of a banaba extract standardized to 1% corosolic acid. After two weeks, their average blood sugar level had dropped by 30%. [2]

Reverses prediabetes. In a study of 10 people with prediabetes (their average glucose level was 104), taking 10 mg of a banaba extract standardized to 198% corosolic acid decreased blood sugar level by an average of 12 points—reversing prediabetes! [4]

Reduces low-grade inflammation. Korean researchers studied 94 people with either prediabetes or diabetes, giving them either an herbal product that included banaba extract or a placebo. After six months, those taking banaba had lower levels of several biomarkers of systemic, low-grade inflammation—which worsens diabetes. [5]

One year later—banaba is still working. In a study of people with prediabetes and diabetes, a year of supplementing with banaba extract lowered blood sugar levels by an average of 16%. [6]

These studies, said Dr. Stohs, show that banaba extract…an extract standardized to corosolic acid (the active ingredient in banaba)…and corosolic acid itself…all work to regulate blood sugar.

In general, banaba lowers blood glucose within two hours of taking the herb, and levels typically go down 10 to 15%.

More good news from Dr. Stohs: there have been no "adverse effects" of banaba in any of the studies, including the study in which people took banaba extract for 1 year.

(Dr. Stohs says there is one published case study that attempted to link kidney damage to corosolic acid—in a diabetes patient who already had kidney damage, and was taking a painkiller known to cause kidney damage. "This is the kind of case study that should never see the light of day," he told me.)

Corosolic acid: an active ingredient that's *very* active

Corosolic acid is the active ingredient of banaba—and it's very active! It can…

- *Activate enzymes* that limit the breakdown and absorption of sugars and starches, which would otherwise turn into glucose.

- *Decrease gluconeogenesis*, the creation of glucose in the liver.

- *Increase GLUT4*—a protein that works with insulin to move glucose into the muscle and fat cells.

- *Activate PPARs* (peroxisome proliferator-activated receptors), which trigger genes that help increase insulin sensitivity.

- *Help cells use blood sugar* so it doesn't linger in the bloodstream.

- *Lower blood fats* that would otherwise clog insulin receptors.

Taking the right dose

The studies showing that banaba works were mostly conducted with banaba extracts…that were standardized to corosolic acid (anywhere from 1% to 18%)…with the study participants taking between 3 to 10 mg of corosolic acid daily.

Dr. Stohs told me that banaba is most likely to be effective taken twice a day, with meals—taking 3 to 5 mg of corosolic acid each time.

For example, one product has capsules containing 250 mg of banaba leaf…standardized to 1.5% corosolic acid…delivering 3 mg of corosolic acid per capsule. According to Dr. Stohs' recommendation, you'd take one capsule, twice a day, with meals.

Dr. Stohs also told me he doesn't think the percentage of corosolic acid matters. That is, there is no scientific evidence showing that a product standardized to 18% corosolic acid is any "stronger" or more effective than a product standardized to 1%. (In fact, the 1% product might be *more* effective, since it would retain more unknown factors in the herb that might also be affecting blood sugar, said Dr. Stohs.)

Many of the studies on banaba were conducted with a soft gel extract that was called Glucosol, and which is now sold under the names GlucoFit and GlucoHelp.

However, those product names aren't what's important. Rather, look for a banaba supplement that meets the criteria specified by Dr. Stohs: standardized to at least 1% corosolic acid…taking 3 to 5 mg of corosolic acid…twice a day…with meals.

Going bananas for banaba

Worldwide, many folks with diabetes have found banaba beneficial:

Glucose control better than ever. "My blood glucose control seems to be better than ever after taking three, 300 mg banaba pills per day, for five days," says a post at http://forum.lowcarber.org. "I am waking up with fasting blood glucose in the low 80s."

Glucose 10 to 20 points lower. "A few weeks ago, I bought a banaba product and took one tablet with my dinner meal," says a post from the same site. "I noticed my fasting blood glucose was lower by 10 to 20 points on average."

Banaba makes a big difference. "I was diagnosed with diabetes in May and have been watching things closely since then," says a post on www.celiac.org. "The banaba makes a big difference, and can lower the blood glucose for me."

Glucose always under 100. "I am a type 2 diabetic and use two alternative products for blood glucose and insulin regulation—cinnamon (500 mgs, twice a day) and banaba (200 mgs, twice a day)," says a post at www.healthexpertadvice.org. My fasting blood glucose is *always* under 100.

Blood glucose: from "way over 200" to 99. "Recently, I chatted with a person who also has type 2 diabetes, and he told me that he had begun taking banaba leaf and that it's helping him control his blood glucose—that his blood glucose is way down," says a post at www.diabeticconnect.com. "He said he's still taking his oral meds, but no insulin! Well, I want to get off my diabetes meds, so I bought some banaba leaf and started taking it three times daily, with meals. (Of course, I am also watching my diet very carefully and I've begun walking.) For the past two days, I have not had to take any meds! Sometimes, before this, my readings have been way over 200, sometimes close to 300—and now they're down to 122 and lower. For instance, 99 today!!!!!!!!"

Anti-diabetes secrets in the next chapter...

• How gymnema may regenerate the insulin-manufacturing beta-cells of the pancreas—essentially, bringing dead cells back to life!

• Not all gymnema is the same: this uniquely powerful extract can lower blood sugar by an astounding 70 to 80 points after six months of use—from the 200s to the 120s or 130s! ("My morning blood sugar was 161 and is now down to 106," says one amazed user.)

• "90 percent of people with type 2 diabetes could be completely normalized" with gymnema extract, says this naturopathic physician.

EXPERTS AND CONTRIBUTORS:

Sid Stohs, PhD, is Dean Emeritus of Creighton University Medical Center in Omaha, Nebraska.

REFERENCES:

1. Stohs, et al. A review of the efficacy and safety of banaba (Lagerstroemia speciosa L.) and corosolic acid. *Phytotherapy Research*, 2012 Mar;26(3):317-24.

2. Fukushima M, et al. Effect of corosolic acid on postchallenge plasma glucose levels. *Diabetes Research and Clinical Practice*, 2006 Aug;73(2):174-7.

3. Judy WV, et al. Antidiabetic activity of a standardized extract (Glucosol) from Lagerstroemia speciosa leaves in Type II diabetics. A dose-dependence study. *Journal of Ethnopharmacology*, 2003 Jul;87(1):115-7.

4. Tsuchibe S, et al. An inhibitory effect on the increase in postprandial glucose by banaba extract capsule enriched corosolic acid. *Journal for the Integrated Study of Dietary Habits*, 17: 255-259.

5. Kim HJ, et al. A six-month supplementation of mulberry, Korean red ginseng, and banaba decreases biomarkers of systemic low-grade inflammation in subjects with impaired glucose tolerance and type 2 diabetes.

6. Ikeda Y, et al. Blood glucose controlling effects and safety of single and long-term administration on the extract of banaba leaves. *Journal of Nutrition and Food*, 5: 41-53.

Chapter 20

Gymnema Sylvestre

Balancing blood sugar for 2,000 years

If your condition is *madhu meha*, then *gumar* is for you.

Translation from the Hindi: If you have "honey urine" (diabetes), you should take "the sugar destroyer" (the herb *gymnema sylvestre*).

At least that's been one of the standard anti-diabetes recommendations for the past 2,000 years from practitioners of Ayurveda, the ancient system of natural healing from India.

Gymnema is a vine-like plant found in the tropical forests of southern and central India, and it has a very unusual effect: chew on the leaves, and you'll temporarily lose your ability to taste sweets! (They don't call it "the sugar destroyer" for nothing.)

Modern science has figured out the molecular interactions underlying this sweet-slaying magic, according to Indian researchers from the University of Mumbai in their whimsically-titled scientific paper, *Gymnema sylvestre: A Memoir*. [1]

The *gymnemic acids* in the herb have a structure similar to glucose (sugar) molecules. First, those molecules "fill the receptor locations on the taste buds," preventing their activation by sugar molecules in food. Next, the gymnemic acids fill up the sugar receptors in the intestine, blocking the absorption of glucose—and lowering blood sugar levels. But they're not done yet.

Gymnemic acids also stimulate (and may even regenerate) the beta-cells of the pancreas that manufacture insulin, the hormone that guides glucose out of the bloodstream and into cells. And the acids rev up enzymes that help the body use glucose.

Figuring out the mechanisms of action of gymnemic acids is all well and good. But what happens when the herb is put to the glucose-controlling test?

Success happens: Two decades of scientific research has confirmed two millennium of gymnema's use—it *is* a powerful herbal treatment for diabetes.

Regenerating the pancreas, reducing blood sugar

Three studies on gymnema were conducted on an extract from gymnema leaves called GS4.

The first study showed that it could regenerate insulin-manufacturing pancreatic cells in diabetic rats. [2]

Then two studies on people, published in the *Journal of Ethnopharmacology*, showed that GS4 worked in both pre-diabetes and diabetes. [3, 4] After four months of daily use of the extract (200 milligrams, 3 times a day), there was a...

- 23% reduction in fasting blood glucose in people with type II diabetes,

- 15% reduction in A1C in people with type II diabetes

- 30% reduction in fasting blood glucose in people with pre-diabetes

In one of the studies, five out of 22 diabetes patients were able to *completely discontinue* their diabetes drugs after taking GS4. (In another study, type 1 diabetes patients taking GS4 were able to reduce their insulin dosages by 14%.)

Since those studies, conducted in 1989 and 1990, the team that first formulated GS4 has refined the extract.

"We continued our work after making GS4 because we knew there was more potential to be tapped," said Michael Baker, ND, a naturopathic physician with clinics in Bellevue and Spokane, Washington. "In 1999 we patented our final and most up-to-date gymnema-based extract, and called it ProBeta, which is more pure, potent and concentrated than GS4. It's easier for the body to process and it works more quickly."

Research shows that ProBeta outperforms GS4 by 42% in lowering blood sugar levels in people with diabetes.

"90% of people with diabetes could be normalized with ProBeta"

"This supplement is amazing—a kind of tonic for the pancreas," Dr. Baker told me. "In the average patient with type 2 diabetes, running glucose levels in the 200s, 2 caps, twice a day, can drop levels down to the 120s or 130s after five to six months of use. If you give 2 caps three times day, you can get levels right at 100 or so. I'd say that 90 percent of the people with type 2 diabetes I've seen could be completely normalized with ProBeta, along with diet, exercise and stress management techniques.

"I had one patient with metabolic syndrome who took 2 capsules, twice a day, for two weeks—and their blood sugar levels fell to the extent that we had to back down to 1 capsule twice a day for two weeks, and then the person eventually got off the supplement because they didn't need it any more."

"It dropped my blood sugar 30 points in two months."

Dr. Baker's experience with his patients is seconded by many other folks taking the supplement…

"I was diagnosed with diabetes 12 years ago and have been on many different prescription drugs," said Sam G. "But I also use natural products that work for me—and the best of them is Pro Beta. It dropped my blood sugar about 30 points after just two months—and I check my blood sugar eight to ten times a day, so I could clearly see it going down. If you have diabetes, you owe it to yourself to try it for a couple of months—and definitely let your doctor know what you have done, because you're probably going to need less medication."

"With ProBeta, my blood sugar has gone from pre-diabetic to healthy levels—even though I'm still eating bad foods," said Dan D.

"My morning blood sugar was 161—and ProBeta has brought it down to 106," said Veronica B. "And I'm not craving sweet foods anymore. *And* my weight is stable. This supplement is working really well for me—and I'm 77 years old."

"I'm not diabetic, but I've had blood sugar issues my entire life, with big ups and downs," said Sharon C. "My doctor wanted to put me on meds but they come with their own set of problems. I tried ProBeta instead and it controlled my sugar swings. This drugless, plant-based approach really gives me comfort."

New research from London

Lately, another gymnema extract has made its way into the pages of medical journals, courtesy of studies conducted by the Diabetes Research Group in the School of Medicine at King's College London. The extract is OSA (Om Shanti Adivasi), named by its Ayurvedic formulator after the Santal tribe in India, which has used gymnema as a folk remedy for centuries. (*Om* is a general term pointing toward the "truth" or effectiveness of the formula; *Adivasi* is a general term for forest-dwelling tribes.)

In a 2012 study of diabetic mice, the extract stimulated the production of insulin and helped the mice handle glucose better. [5] In another 2012 study, using pancreatic cells from mice and humans, OSA triggered the cells to secrete more insulin. [6] And in a study on people with diabetes, taking 1,000 mg of the extract daily for two months lowered fasting blood glucose and post-meal blood glucose. [7]

"OSA may provide a potential alternative therapy for the hyperglycemia [high blood sugar] associated with type 2 diabetes," concluded the scientists in *Phytotherapy Research*.

OSA is sold in the U.S. as the supplement Assurance Blood Health Support.

"I am very impressed with Assurance Blood Health Support," said Kari U., a wellness professional. "Two of my clients did a four-week trial period taking the supplement daily—with great success in controlling blood sugar levels. They were thrilled and so were their doctors."

The recommended dosage is one capsule, two to three times daily.

Reliably standardized products

Natural Standard—a company that generates comprehensive scientific reports (monographs) on natural remedies—says the following supplements are reliably standardized for gymnemic acids, as verified by a third party:

• ProBeta, from PharmaTerra

• Beta Fast GXR, from Informulab

• Gymnesyl, from Nature's Herbs

• Gymnema, from Nature's Way

"My go-to herb for folks with high blood sugar"

One health practitioner who has had great success using gymnema (and other anti-diabetes herbs and supplements) with his clients is Michael Gaeta, LAc, a clinical nutritionist, herbalist and acupuncturist, with private practices in Colorado and New York.

"It is my go-to herb for folks with patterns of high blood sugar, as well as folks with sweet cravings," he told me. "Using gymnema and an overall program for controlling diabetes, I've treated insulin-dependent people with type 2 diabetes who have been able to reduce their need for insulin by 30 to 40%. It is *the* key herb for diabetes patients. It's also key for people with sugar cravings—it's like willpower in a bottle."

The optimal dosage of gymnema is 400 mg, three times a day, with food, because the herb "works quickly to reduce glucose uptake from food," he said.

Gaeta favors gymnema from MediHerb, which is available in the U.S. from health practitioners who sell Standard Process supplements. (Standard Process—which sells whole food rather than synthetic supplements—does not sell directly to consumers. To find a health practitioner who uses Standard Process products, see the Resources section at the end of the chapter.)

Another Standard Process supplement Gaeta uses to treat diabetes is Diaplex, which includes chromium, magnesium and other nutrients featured in this Special Report. "I recently saw a client who had a fasting glucose level of 300—a level that should be below 90. I started her on Diaplex, which she took daily for the following week, until our next visit; she didn't change her diet or exercise or do anything else different. At the next visit, her fasting blood sugar had dropped 150 points.

"With gymnema from MediHerb, Diaplex and other natural treatments I have had 100% success rate with lowering blood sugar in diabetes patients."

To *prevent* blood sugar imbalances as you age, Gaeta favors the product HerbaVital, from MediHerb. "This product is a formulation from the master herbalist Kerry Bone, founder of MediHerb," said Gaeta. "It contains five herbs that are key in preventing or reversing insulin resistance, the imbalance in blood sugar regulation that is the underlying cause of diabetes, heart disease, obesity, and Alzheimer's. It's an all-purpose herbal for anybody over 40 to prevent the common diseases of aging and enjoy robust health."

(The herbs in the formula are Japanese Knotweed root, a superb source of resveratrol; pine bark; milk thistle; Korean ginseng; and ginkgo biloba.)

Anti-diabetes secrets in the next chapter...

- Apple cider vinegar is a classic home remedy, but only one use is SCIENCE-PROVEN: blood sugar control!

- The stunning results of university-based apple cider vinegar studies: lower insulin resistance...lower post-meal glucose levels...more effective than diabetes drugs...and long-term blood sugar control.

- Six key tips for putting more vinegar in your diet.

EXPERTS AND CONTRIBUTORS:

Michael Baker, ND, is a homeopathic and naturopathic physician with clinics in Bellevue and Spokane, Washington.
Website: www.wahomeopathy.com

Michael Gaeta, LAc, is a clinical nutritionist, herbalist and acupuncturist, with private practices in Boulder, Colorado, Forest Hills, New York and Huntington, New York.
Website: www.gaetacommunications.com
Twitter: @michaelcgaeta
Facebook: https://www.facebook.com/gaetacommunications
YouTube Channel: http://www.youtube.com/user/GaetaCommunications/feed

RESOURCES:

To order ProBeta:
Website: www.pharmaterra.com

To order Blood Assurance Health Support:
Website: www.santalsolutions.com, which provides links to many online retailers that sell the product, and also a "store locator" to find a store near you that sells it.

To find a health practitioner near you who sells Standard Process and MediHerb products:
Website: www.standardprocess.com, which has a "Find a Doctor" function on their homepage.

For more information about Natural Standard, a company that provides evidence-based information on natural remedies:
Website: www.naturalstandard.com

REFERENCES:

1. Kanetkar P, et al. Gymnema sylvestre: A Memoir. *Journal of Clinical Biochemistry and Nutrition*. September 2007, 41, 77-81.

2. Shanmugasundaram ER, et al. Possible regeneration of the islets of Langerhans in streptozotocin-diabetic rats given Gymnema sylvestre leaf extracts. *Journal of Ethnopharmacology*, 1990;30:265-279.

3. Baskaran K, et al. Antidiabetic effect of a leaf extract from Gymnema sylvestre in non-insulin-dependent diabetes mellitus patients. *Journal of Ethnopharmacology*, 1990;30:295-305.

4. Shanmugasundaram ER, et al. Use of Gymnema sylvestre leaf extract in the control of blood glucose in insulin-dependent diabetes mellitus. *Journal of Ethnopharmacology*, 1990;30(3):281-294.

5. Al-Romaiyan A, et al. A Novel Extract of Gymnema sylvestre Improves Glucose Tolerance In Vivo and Stimulates Insulin Secretion In Vitro. *Phytotherapy Research*, August 21, 2012.

6. Al-Romaiyan, et al. Investigation of intracellular signaling cascades mediating stimulatory effect of Gymnema sylvestre extract on insulin secretion from isolated mouse and human islets of Langerhans. *Diabetes, Obesity and Metabolism*, July 2012, 6;9999(9999)

7. Al-Romaiyan A, et al. A novel Gymnema sylvestre extract stimulates insulin secretion from human islets in vivo and in vitro. *Phytotherapy Research*, September 2010;24(9):1370-6.

PART V

Anti-Diabetes Super-foods

Dig in and heal.

Chapter 21

Apple Cider Vinegar

This classic home remedy can remedy diabetes, too.

I owe a lot to apple cider vinegar.

In 2000, my then-new book *Alternative Cures* was looking like a flop. Advertising copywriters had tried three approaches to selling the book, and all three had failed. Then they created an advertisement with the headline, <u>Melt Away Artery Plaque—with Apple Cider Vinegar!</u>—and the book started selling like gangbusters in the US and abroad.

Alternative Cures went on to sell more than a million copies.

Yes, people love to read about (and use) apple cider vinegar, the classic home remedy. One book's A-to-Z of vinegar remedies runs for 20 pages, starting with acne, age spots and arthritis (not to mention, *ants repelled*), continuing through headaches, heart disease and hiccups (and *heavily soiled hands*), and wrapping up with sinusitis, toothaches and weight loss (and *wrapping tape adheres better*).

But if you enter the key words "apple cider vinegar" into the massive medical database of scientific studies maintained by the National Institutes of Health, you'll find <u>only one disease with credible, consistent, scientific *proof* for the healing power of apple cider vinegar in people—and that disease is type 2 diabetes.</u>

Four remarkable studies on vinegar and diabetes

To find out more about using apple cider vinegar to beat diabetes, I called Carol Johnston, PhD, RD, a professor of nutrition and director of the nutrition program in the School of Nutrition and Health Promotion at Arizona State University. Dr. Johnston has conducted four studies and published nine scientific papers on the topic, so she knows whereof she speaks.

How did she become interested in using apple cider vinegar for diabetes? I asked her.

"I was conducting research on lower-carb, higher-protein diets for diabetes, like the Atkins Diet and the Zone Diet," she told me. "And, yes, those diets do help control glucose levels. But they also require making major changes in how you eat. The people participating in my studies couldn't *wait* until the studies were over. They found dietary adherence difficult, and certainly didn't intend to keep eating that way after the study—even though their glucose and insulin numbers had improved.

"Coincidentally, while reviewing the scientific research on nutrition for diabetes, I came across a study from the 1980s in which researchers added vinegar to the chow of diabetic rats and were able to control their glycemic response—the increase in blood sugar after eating.

"I said to myself, 'Well, if all you have to do is add vinegar to the diet to control blood sugar, that's a whole lot easier than what I'm trying to make people do by eating these hard-to-follow diets.'"

So Dr. Johnston set out to research the use of apple cider vinegar to control diabetes—and ended up conducting four studies over the next few years.

Before I describe those studies, however, I'd like to take a moment to talk about the *many* varieties of vinegar. You can make vinegar from any carbohydrate that's capable of being fermented. There's also balsamic vinegar, made from white grapes…other fruit vinegars, like raspberry…coconut vinegar, used extensively in Southeast Asian cuisine…rice vinegar…wine vinegar, made from white or red wine…and on and on. Some but not all of the scientific studies I'm about to report did use apple cider vinegar. But, as you'll read later in the chapter, *any* dietary vinegar can work to improve blood sugar control. Now back to the studies.

2004: Vinegar lowers insulin resistance by 64%. Dr. Johnston studied 31 people—10 were healthy; 11 had insulin resistance; and 10 had type 2 diabetes. She divided them into two groups.

One group downed a drink consisting of two tablespoons of apple cider vinegar in water, with a little saccharine; the other downed a placebo drink.

Two minutes later, both groups ate a meal consisting of a buttered, white flour bagel and a glass of orange juice—delivering a hefty 87 grams of carbohydrate.

Thirty and 60 minutes after the meal, she measured their blood glucose and insulin levels.

One week later, she conducted the same experiment, with the original apple cider group drinking the placebo this time, and the placebo group drinking the vinegar.

Results: In those who were insulin resistant, insulin sensitivity (the ability to use the hormone) was improved by 34% when they drank vinegar before meals; insulin sensitivity was also improved by 19% in people with type 2 diabetes.

Vinegar also lowered postprandial glycemia (the post-meal spikes in blood sugar linked to the advance of diabetes and to heart disease)—by 64% among the insulin resistant; and by 17% in people with diabetes.

Those findings are particularly important if you have insulin resistance or prediabetes— because increasing your insulin sensitivity might stop your condition from developing into diabetes, Dr. Johnston told me.

"Further investigations to examine the efficacy of vinegar as an anti-diabetic therapy are warranted," she wrote in *Diabetes Care*. And so she kept investigating…

2005: Vinegar lowers post-meal glucose levels by 55%. Dr. Johnston conducted her second study on 11 healthy people, who ate a high-carb meal and then drank vinegar. Once again, vinegar reduced post-meal glucose levels by 55%, compared to those not drinking it.

"…the addition of vinegar…to a high-glycemic load meal significantly reduced postprandial [post-meal] glycemia," she wrote in *Diabetes Care*. [2] (This is great news for healthy folks who want to prevent diabetes.)

2007: Vinegar may work better than diabetes drugs. For her next experiment, Dr. Johnston studied 11 people with type 2 diabetes, giving them 2 tablespoons of apple cider vinegar at bedtime.

The next morning, fasting glucose levels were 6% lower—compared to only 0.7% lower on mornings when the participants didn't use vinegar the night before. [3]

Six percent may not sound like much. But these were folks who had been diagnosed with diabetes only a few years before, and whose diabetes was well-controlled. Medications for similar diabetes patients typically lower fasting glucose by 3 to 6%—so vinegar worked just as well, if not better, than diabetes drugs!

"Vinegar is widely available, it is affordable, and it is appealing as a remedy," wrote Dr. Johnston in *Diabetes Care*.

2009: Vinegar lowers A1C, a measure of long-term glucose control. Next, Dr. Johnston studied 27 people with type 2 diabetes, giving them either vinegar, vinegar pills or pickles (which are very vinegary). Only the vinegar lowered A1C.

"Regular vinegar use…improved glycemic control," she wrote, in *Diabetes Research and Clinical Practice*. [4]

2010: Conclusion—vinegar works! In her most recent scientific paper on vinegar, Dr. Johnston summarized the findings of her four studies—and concluded that two tablespoons of vinegar, taken right before a meal of complex carbohydrates (like bread, potatoes, pasta or rice), reduces post-meal blood sugar levels by an average of 20% more than a placebo, in people with diabetes and in healthy people. [5]

"The antiglycemic properties of vinegar are evident," she wrote in *Annals of Nutrition & Metabolism*. A lot of other scientists agree with her.

Worldwide support for the power of vinegar

Dr. Johnston isn't the only scientist studying vinegar and diabetes—research has been conducted by scientists around the globe. Standout scientific findings include…

Greece: People with diabetes can eat potatoes—if they use vinegar, too. Researchers in Greece studied 16 people with type 2 diabetes, measuring post-meal glucose levels after a high-carb meal of mashed potatoes. When the diabetes patients used vinegar, their average blood glucose level was 181; when they didn't use vinegar, it was 311—a huge difference. [6]

Sweden: Ditto on the potatoes for healthy folks. Researchers in Sweden conducted a study on 13 healthy people—and found that using a vinaigrette dressing (vinegar and olive oil) on a meal of potatoes reduced post-meal glucose levels by 43% and post-meal insulin levels by 31%, compared to eating potatoes without the dressing. [7]

Japan: Vinegar for the metabolic syndrome. In a Japanese study, daily intake of vinegar for three months lowered weight, reduced belly fat and lowered triglycerides in people with the metabolic syndrome. "Daily intake of vinegar might be useful in the prevention of metabolic syndrome," concluded the researchers. [8]

Middle East: Vinegar reduces the chronic inflammation that drives diabetes. In a small study of diabetes patients, researchers from the Middle East found that three months of using vinegar lowered biomarkers of chronic inflammation—which many health experts think is the main problem driving both diabetes and heart disease. [9]

"There is an accumulating amount of scientific literature from multiple labs all over the world showing the same thing—that vinegar works to balance blood sugar and insulin levels," Dr. Johnston told me. "I feel confident that the anti-diabetic action of vinegar is a real phenomenon."

How vinegar works to balance blood sugar

Okay, vinegar works. But *how* does it work?

Based on the evidence, Dr. Johnston thinks that the *acetic acid* in vinegar (the compound that gives vinegar its tart flavor and pungent odor) blunts the activity of *disaccharidase* enzymes (sucrase, lactase, maltase), which help break down complex carbs, like those in potatoes, rice, bread and pasta.

As a result, those foods are digested and absorbed more slowly, lowering blood glucose and insulin levels.

In other words, vinegar interferes with the digestion of starches—making it a perfect super-food for people with blood sugar problems.

The acetic acid test: Most doctors don't pass it

But don't bother asking your doctor about the starch-taming power of vinegar. It's likely he won't know a thing about it.

"The medical profession doesn't seem to have any interest in vinegar for diabetes—in fact, most doctors have never even heard of it," Dr. Johnston said. "I have people emailing me all the time, saying, 'My doctor doesn't know about this, so can you tell me what I need to know to lower my blood sugar with vinegar.'

"And there's a similar lack of interest from the American Diabetes Association. Based on the very positive results of my research, I was hoping they would fund a larger study, but they haven't.

"And most diabetes researchers aren't paying attention, either. For example, the Mediterranean diet is one of the best diets for diabetes control, and it's also the diet with the highest content of vinegar. I remember sitting next to a big proponent of the Mediterranean diet at a scientific conference and saying, 'It's the *vinegar* in the diet that's probably making the difference for diabetes'—but he didn't buy it."

Fortunately, you don't have to wait for your doctor, the American Diabetes Association or a Nobel laureate to give you permission to use vinegar to control blood sugar.

And using vinegar is incredibly easy…

Vinegar as mealtime medicine: Two tablespoons is all it takes

Here are lots of ways to use vinegar to stop a post-meal rise in glucose and insulin after a starchy meal…

Use two tablespoons. That's the amount that worked in all of Dr. Johnston's studies. More isn't more effective, she said.

Put it in a salad dressing. The ideal ratio is two tablespoons of vinegar to one part oil. Any kind of oil is fine, from olive to canola. And so is any kind of vinegar. ("I favor the wine vinegars," said Dr. Johnston. "They're smoother, with less bite.") Add some favorite seasonings to make the dressing more tasty.

If you use a commercial vinaigrette from a bottle as a dressing, add an additional tablespoon of vinegar to each serving.

Eat the salad first. (Or otherwise consume the vinegar early in the meal.) You want the acetic acid to disrupt the carb-digesting enzymes *before* they have a chance to get to work.

Another way to get your vinegar early in the meal is to dip pre-meal bread in a vinaigrette dressing. (Remember: *two* parts vinegar to *one* part oil.)

Use plenty of mustard. "For instance, if you a eat a big sandwich, go heavy on the mustard—which is basically a vinegar-rich condiment," Dr. Johnston said.

Try a commercial apple cider vinegar drink. Dr. Johnston's studies used Organic Apple Cider Vinegar All-Natural Drinks, from Bragg. They come in several flavors, including Apple-Cinnamon, Concord Grape-Acai, Ginger Spice, Limeade and Sweet Stevia. Just down the drink as an appetizer—and dig in!

"My study participants became true believers in this product," Dr. Johnson told me.

(For ordering information, see the Resources section at the end of the chapter.)

Use vinegar only for starchy meals. Vinegar only works on *starches*—bread, rice, pasta and potatoes. You can't down a can of soda with a vinegar chaser and expect the vinegar to stop a quick rise in blood sugar

Enjoy! "I always use vinegar with my evening meals, and go through about a bottle a week," Dr. Johnston told me. "It's such a fun solution to preventing or controlling blood sugar problems!"

Anti-diabetes secrets in the next chapter...

- Startling new scientific finding from the University of Washington: Kidney disease is the #1 risk factor for death in people with diabetes.

- This four-year study shows that increasing your daily intake of *soy foods* can REVERSE diabetic kidney disease—a result so remarkable scientists were shaking their heads. (They were sure the patients in their study would get worse.)

- The perfect "prescription" for the amount of daily soy food that protects kidneys.

- How to use baking soda—yes, *baking soda*—to prevent kidney failure.

EXPERTS AND CONTRIBUTORS:

Carol Johnston, PhD, RD, is a professor of nutrition and director of the nutrition program in the School of Nutrition and Health Promotion at Arizona State University.

RESOURCES:

To order Organic Apple Cider Vinegar All-Natural Drinks, from Bragg:
Go to the webpage:
http://bragg.com/products/bragg-organic-healthy-live-food-products.html
Or call: **800-446-1990**

REFERENCES:

1. Johnston, CS, et al. Vinegar Improves Insulin Sensitivity to a High-Carbohydrate Meal in Subjects With Insulin Resistance or Type 2 Diabetes. *Diabetes Care*, Volume 27, Number 1, January 2004, Pgs. 281-282.

2. Johnston CS, et al. Vinegar and peanut products as complementary foods to reduce postprandial glycemia. *Journal of the American Dietetic Association*, 2005 Dec;105(12):1939-42.

3. White AM, et al. Vinegar Ingestion at Bedtime Moderates Waking Glucose Concentrations in Adults with Well-Controlled Type 2 Diabetes. *Diabetes Care*, Volume 30, Number 11, November 2007, pgs. 2814-2815.

4. Johnston CS, et al. Preliminary evidence that regular vinegar ingestion favorably influences hemoglobin A1C values in individuals with type 2 diabetes mellitus. *Diabetes Research and Clinical Practice*, 2009 May;84(2).

5. Johnston CS, et al. Examination of the antiglycemic properties of vinegar in healthy adults. *Annals of Nutrition & Metabolism*, 2010;56(1):74-9.

6. Liatis S, et al. Vinegar reduces postprandial hyperglycaemia in patients with type II diabetes when added to a high, but not to a low, glycaemic index meal.

7. Leeman M, et al. Vinegar dressing and cold storage of potatoes lowers postprandial glycaemic and insulinaemic responses in healthy subjects. *European Journal of Clinical Nutrition*, 2005 Nov;59(11):1266-71.

8. Kondo T, et al. Vinegar intake reduces body weight, body fat mass, and serum triglyceride levels in obese Japanese subjects. *Bioscience, Biotechnology and Biochemistry*, 2009 Aug;73(8):1837-43.

9. Golazarand, M. Effects of processed Berberis vulgaris in apple vinegar on blood pressure and inflammatory markers in type 2 diabetic patients. *Journal of Diabetes and Metabolic Disorders*, 2008;7:3.

Chapter 22

Soy Foods

They can protect weakened kidneys—and help keep you alive.

Diabetes dramatically increases the risk of heart disease—and it's heart disease that's the #1 killer of diabetes patients.

I've written that sentence or one like it many times, in many articles and books (including this one)—because that's what diabetes experts have always told me.

But new research out of the University of Washington in Seattle and Spokane—published one month before I finished writing this Special Report—presented a startlingly different set of facts.

Kidney disease, claimed the study's researchers, is the #1 risk factor for death in people with diabetes.

"We've all been trained to think of type 2 diabetes as a bad thing—but it's particularly bad when you get kidney disease, too," said Maryam Afkarian, MD, PhD, a kidney specialist and assistant professor of medicine at the Kidney Research Institute at the University of Washington School of Medicine. [1]

Dr. Afkarian and her colleagues analyzed 10 years of health data from more than 15,000 people. In terms of understanding *why* people with diabetes die, their results were revolutionary.

First, they learned that 42% of people with diabetes have kidney disease, compared to only 9% of those without diabetes.

Next, they discovered that people with diabetes who didn't have kidney disease had a 10-year death rate of 11%—over the years of the study, 11 out of 100 died.

But those with diabetes *and* kidney disease had a much higher death rate—31%! For those diabetes patients, the risk of dying was nearly *triple* that of diabetes patients without kidney disease!

"Those with kidney disease predominantly account for the increased mortality observed in type 2 diabetes," the researchers wrote in the *Journal of the American Society of Nephrology*. [2]

In other words, most people who die from diabetes die because of kidney disease!

"It was surprising that kidney disease was such a prominent marker of dying early in type 2 diabetes," said Dr. Afkarian. [3]

Important fact: *Kidney disease* in diabetes (diabetic nephropathy) is so deadly mainly because it worsens the risk of *heart disease*, point out the researchers. That fact will take on added importance later in the chapter, when I introduce you to the dietary solution to this problem, which protects and strengthens the kidneys *and* the heart.

"We should focus on preventing kidney disease from developing in people with diabetes— and if they do develop it, we should try to slow it down," said Dr. Afkarian. [3]

Dr. Afkarian and other kidney specialists at the University of Washington make several commonsense medical and lifestyle recommendations for the 42% of diabetes patients who already have kidney disease, such as: controlling blood sugar; controlling blood pressure with ACE inhibitors or angiotensin receptor blocker, medications that also protect the kidneys; taking medications that protect the kidneys from excess protein; taking medication to lower cholesterol, if needed; avoiding medications that can hurt the kidneys, like non-steroidal anti-inflammatory drugs such as ibuprofen; losing weight; exercising regularly; and stopping smoking.

But there's a kidney-protecting action-item that's not among their recommendations—a specific dietary strategy that a recent four-year study shows may not only *stop* but also *reverse* diabetic nephropathy.

Eat more soy foods!

Kidneys 101

But before we talk about how soy can protect your kidneys, let's take a moment to understand exactly what your kidneys do—and how diabetes damages them. To better understand the kidneys—bean-shaped, fist-sized organs on either side of the spine at the back of the abdominal cavity, below the ribcage—I talked with Katherine Tuttle, MD, clinical professor of medicine in the Kidney Research Institute at the University of Washington School of Medicine, and one of the authors of the new study on the dangers of kidney disease.

Kidneys contain millions of tiny blood vessels—the *glomeruli*—that filter and clean the blood, she explained. But that's not all kidneys do. They manufacture hormones that regulate blood pressure…maintain the body's acid-alkaline balance…and produce a form of vitamin D that strengthens bones. "They are absolutely essential to health—and it is essential that you maintain their function," she said.

But diabetes can destroy your kidneys. In fact, diabetes is the most common cause of kidney failure, accounting for more than 50% of all cases in the U.S.

That's because high levels of blood sugar force the kidneys to work harder, damaging their delicate filters. Year by year, your *glomerular filtration rate* (GFR)—a measurement of how much blood passes through the glomeruli—decreases. A healthy level is 100 to 140; when it's lower than 60 for at least three months, you are diagnosed with kidney disease. (Anyone with diabetes should have a GFR test as part of their annual physical, said Dr. Tuttle. "But the rate of physicians performing this test is woefully low, with less than half of people with diabetes receiving it.") The damaged filters also allow more protein (albumin) in your urine.

To complicate matters, kidney disease doesn't produce any symptoms until the kidneys are about to fail. And when they do fail, the only treatments are a kidney transplant or dialysis, the regular filtering of blood with a machine.

But enough bad news about your kidneys. Let's talk about the good news: soy foods.

Soy: super-food for weakened kidneys and threatened hearts

Dozens of scientific studies show that soy is a nutritional ally for diabetes patients with kidney disease.

But the best (and one of the most recent) of these studies, published in *Diabetes Care*, shows that eating lots of soy can help *reverse* signs of kidney disease and risk factors for heart disease—and lower blood sugar, too! [4]

And remember: kidney disease kills many diabetes patients by worsening heart disease—so any food that can handle kidney disease *and* heart disease is definitely a super-food for diabetes.

Here's the study…

After years of eating a high-soy diet—healthier kidneys and healthier hearts. The four-year study involved 41 diabetes patients with kidney disease. They were divided into two groups. One group ate a diet with protein from 70% animal and 30% vegetable sources. The other group ate a diet with protein from 35% animal sources, 35% textured soy protein, and 30% vegetable proteins. (To present the results, I'll call the 70% animal protein group the "meat group" and the 35% soy protein group the "soy group.")

The soy group had…

<u>A reduction in levels of proteinuria, a biomarker of weakened kidneys.</u> After four years, the soy group's levels were seven times lower than the meat group's.

A reduction in levels of creatinine, another biomarker of kidney disease. At the end of the study, the soy group's levels were three times lower than the meat group's.

Lower fasting blood sugar. The soy group saw an average *decrease* of 18 points. The meat group saw an *increase* of 11 points.

Lower bad LDL cholesterol. The soy group's LDL plunged by 20 points. The meat group's rose by 6.

Lower total cholesterol. The soy group had a drop of 23 points, while the meat group had a rise of 10 points.

Lower triglycerides. The soy group fell by 24 points—five times more than the meat group's.

Lower C-reactive protein, a biomarker for chronic inflammation. The soy group had a drop four times greater than the meat group.

The results are nothing short of amazing—because the researchers expected the kidneys of everybody in the study would get *worse*, even those eating lots of soy.

"As diabetic nephropathy is a progressive disease, we expected the conditions of these patients would have gotten worse after 4 years," they wrote in *Diabetes Care*. "But because of medical and dietary control, their conditions improved."

And you don't have to wait four years for that type of improvement.

In a smaller experiment by the same researchers who conducted the four-year study, a diet rich in soy protein reduced four biomarkers of kidney disease—in just seven weeks! [6]

How does soy protect your kidneys?

There are a lot of opinions out there.

The scientists who conducted the four year study think it works by lowering cholesterol and triglycerides, citing research that links high blood fats to diabetic nephropathy.

Other researchers speculate that substituting soy protein for animal protein eases stress on the filters of the kidney.

Others say that components of soy itself—specifically, its peptides (short chains of amino acids, the building blocks of protein) and isoflavones (estrogen-like plant compounds)—may improve kidney function.

In his scientific paper, *Beneficial effects of soy protein consumption for renal function*, James Anderson, MD, emeritus professor of medicine and clinical nutrition at the University of Kentucky (and an esteemed colleague who I've interviewed many times about soy), says there are three main ways soy helps the kidneys. [5] Soy…

1. Stops the overproduction of *mesangial cells* within the glomeruli, which muck up the filters.

2. Boosts the production of nitric oxide, a compound that improves blood flow in the kidneys (and throughout the body).

3. Normalizes the movement of electrolytes (minerals) within the loop of Henle, a structure in the glomeruli, improving filtration.

We'll leave it to the nephrologists—the kidney experts—to figure all that out. Right now, your questions are probably, How the heck do I get more soy foods into my diet? Do I have to eat…what's that white, tasteless stuff called…*tofu*?

Never fear: you don't have to eat tofu (unless you like it). There are lots of tasty, easy ways to eat more soy.

The soy protein prescription: 16 grams a day

The diabetes patients in the four-year study ate 16 grams of soy protein a day—the amount in two servings of soy foods. And they *substituted* those foods for a portion of their daily animal proteins.

The Soyfoods Association of America provides a webpage that shows grams of protein in specific soy foods; you'll find the URL for that page in the Resources section at the end of the chapter. (However, to be absolutely certain about the grams of protein you're getting from a serving of soy food, check the nutrition label.) Some examples…

Just one soy burger provides 13 grams of soy protein. A bag of soy chips, 7 grams. A cup of soy milk over your morning cereal, 6 grams. A quarter-cup of soy nuts, 11 grams. One-half cup of cooked soy pasta, 13 grams. One-half cup of edamame (my favorite way to get soy) 11 grams. (To make this dish—popular in Japan—steam soybeans for five minutes in their pods, remove the pods, and eat the beans. It's a great appetizer or snack.)

And then, of course, there's always tofu, the bean curd made by pressing the coagulated curds of soy juice into soft, white blocks. Eating a plain chunk of tofu is about as appetizing as eating cotton. But it can provide wonderful texture to stir-fry vegetables, whole grains and other dishes, I was told by Nancy Chapman, RD, executive director of the Soyfoods Association of

North America, who says to use "firm" or "extra-firm" varieties for the best culinary experience.

Want to make a straightforward, soy-for-meat substitution? You'll find a nearly limitless variety of soy substitutes for meat, including soy patties, links and deli slices, said Chapman. (And don't forget the soy cheese.)

A smart strategy: Soy protein powder

A super-simple and science-verified way to meet your daily requirement of soy protein: use isolated soy protein powder.

Scientists in the Division of Nutritional Sciences at the University of Illinois studied 14 men with type 2 diabetes and kidney disease. They asked the men to take soy protein in the form of vanilla-flavored *isolated soy protein powder*, mixed with water, juice or food. After two months of soy, the men had an average 9.5 point drop in urinary levels of albumin. [7]

"This was a very significant clinical result," I was told by John W. Erdman, Jr., PhD, a professor of nutrition at the University of Illinois. Dr. Erdman and his colleagues had hypothesized that isolated soy protein powder might *stop* the rise in albumin but not *reverse* it.

There are many types of soy protein powder on the market, but *isolated soy protein powder* was the type used in the study. The exact type: Supro, from Solae. Two widely available Supro-containing products are: 1) NOW Foods Soy Protein Isolate and 2) SciFit Soy Protein Isolate. They are offered in a variety of flavors, including vanilla, chocolate and strawberry.

For results that match those in his study, Dr. Erdman suggests using 2 grams of powder per 9 pounds of body weight—for example, if you weigh 180 pounds, use 40 grams a day. (Divide body weight by 9 and multiply by 2.)

Divide the dose between two meals, he suggested, with 20 grams at breakfast and 20 grams at lunch. You could mix the powder with a glass of juice in the morning and a cup of yogurt at lunch.

Another surprising natural kidney remedy: Baking Soda

Although this chapter is all about soy, I'd feel remiss if I didn't tell you about an amazingly simple and effective drugless remedy that I encountered while researching diabetic nephropathy. Here's what I found…

Diabetes patients with kidney disease are very susceptible to a condition called *acidosis*—which can happen when kidneys are weak…waste products loiter in the body…and blood chemistry becomes acidic. Acidosis erodes bones, hobbles the immune system, strains the heart, and even further injures the kidneys, pushing them faster toward failure, or end-stage renal disease.

But researchers in the UK found a simple way to control acidosis: Baking soda (sodium bicarbonate).

In a study reported in the *Journal of the American Society of Nephrology*, the researchers studied 134 people with advanced kidney disease and acidosis. They found that adding a daily tablet of sodium bicarbonate to standard treatment dramatically slowed the disease.

Those taking baking soda had kidneys that were 69% more effective at cleaning the blood of *creatinine*, an acidic waste product.

And only 9% of those taking baking soda had "rapid progression" of their kidney disease, compared with 45% of those who didn't take baking soda.

Finally, only 6.5% of those taking the baking soda progressed to end-stage renal disease, compared with 33% of those who didn't take sodium bicarbonate. [8]

The researchers note that taking baking soda didn't trigger higher blood pressure or more water retention—possible side effects from the sodium in sodium bicarbonate.

"This cheap and simple strategy has potential benefits in quality of life and clinical outcome in patients with chronic kidney disease," said Magdi Yaqoob, MD, the study leader.

"While we would want to see several studies replicating these results before routinely recommending baking soda to patients with diabetes and kidney disease, these are remarkably positive findings," Dr. Tuttle told me.

Doctors already routinely treat acidosis in patients with kidney disease, but they do so with medication such as sodium citrate, which converts to sodium bicarbonate in the body. She advises talking to your doctor to see if baking soda might be the right treatment for you.

"It's a therapy that is simple, easily available and cheap, compared with conventional medicines used to treat acidosis," she told me. "You just have to learn exactly how much works in your case, and how to measure it carefully for the effective dosage. You also have to be tested regularly for possible side effects, such as increased blood pressure and fluid retention."

Anti-diabetes secrets in the next chapter...

• All about "resistant starch"—the little-known form of starch that *lowers* blood sugar!

• Scientific evidence that resistant starch can improve insulin sensitivity…stop blood sugar from spiking after meals…and help you burn fat and lose weight.

• Easy ways to put more resistant starch in your diet.

EXPERTS AND CONTRIBUTORS:

James Anderson, MD, is emeritus professor of medicine and clinical nutrition at the University of Kentucky

Maryam Afkarian, MD, PhD, is an assistant professor of medicine in the Division of Nephrology, Kidney Research Institute, at the University of Washington School of Medicine in Seattle.

Nancy Chapman, RD, is the executive director of the Soyfoods Association of North America.

John W. Erdman, Jr., PhD, is a professor of nutrition at the University of Illinois.

Katherine R. Tuttle, MD, is clinical professor of medicine in the Division of Nephrology, Kidney Research Institute, at the University of Washington School of Medicine, and executive director for research at Providence Sacred Heart Medical Center and Children's Hospital.

RESOURCES:

To find out how many grams of protein are in soyfoods:

See this page at the website of the Soyfoods Association of North America:

http://www.soyfoods.org/nutrition-health/soy-for-healthy-living/soy-for-heart-disease/soy-protein-content-chart

REFERENCES:

1. HealthDay, January 24, 2013

http://consumer.healthday.com/Article.asp?AID=672811

2. Afkarian M, et al. Kidney disease and increased mortality risk in type 2 diabetes, *Journal of the American Society of Nephrology*, 2013 Feb;24(2);302-8.

3. Medscape Medical News, January 24, 2013 www.medscape.com/viewarticle/778133

4. Azadbakht, L et al. Soy Protein Intake, Cardiorenal Indices, and C-Reactive Protein in Type 2 Diabetes With Nephropathy. *Diabetes Care*, Volume 31, Number 4, April 2008, Pages 648-654.

5. Anderson, JW. Beneficial effects of soy protein consumption for renal function. *Asia Pacific Journal of Clinical Nutrition*, 2008; 17(SI):324-328.

6. Azadbakht L, et al. Soy-protein consumption and kidney-related biomarkers among type 2 diabetics: a crossover, randomized clinical trial. *Journal of Renal Nutrition,* 2009 Nov;19(6):479-86.

7. Teixeira SR, et al. Isolated soy protein consumption reduces urinary albumin excretion and improves the serum lipid profile in men with type 2 diabetes mellitus and nephropathy. *Journal of Nutrition*, 2004;134-:1874-80.

8. de Brito-Ashurst, I, et al. Bicarbonate supplementation slow progression of CKD and improves nutritional status. *Journal of the American Society of Nephrology*, 2009 Sep;20(9):2075-84.

Chapter 23

Resistant Starch

The carb that doesn't misbehave

Starch is the *enemy* of balanced blood sugar, right?

Starch is the King of Carbs. It's potatoes and bread and rice and pasta and corn. Starch is glucose on steroids, hell-bent on sending blood sugar skyrocketing.

So why would I include a chapter on starch in this Special Report? How could I possibly think that *starch* is a diabetes *super-food*?

Because I talked to Rhonda. Let me explain…

The surprising story of resistant starch

I ran into Rhonda Witwer at Natural Products Expo West, a yearly trade show for the supplement and natural foods industry. She was standing in front of the booth for the company National Starch Food Innovation (now called Ingredion), under a sign boldly proclaiming the glucose-balancing benefits of something called *resistant starch*—something I'd vaguely heard of.

And since I was attending the show for the express purpose of finding the latest, greatest supplements and super-foods to include in this Special Report, I stopped to talk, telling Rhonda who I was, what I was up to—and asking her, What the heck is *resistant starch*?

I'll let Rhonda take it from here…

"Resistant starch has been around for thousands of years," she told me. "It's found in foods like beans, peas, whole grains and bananas that are slightly green. It's also formed when starch-containing foods are cooked and cooled, like potato salad and sushi rice.

"It's called *resistant* because—unlike other starches—it 'resists' being completely digested and absorbed in the small intestine. Instead, quite a bit of it continues down the digestive tract into the large intestine, or colon. There, it acts just like dietary fiber—it's broken down by friendly colonic bacteria, a process that produces a wide variety of health benefits." (Hang around for a minute, and you'll learn all about them.)

"Unfortunately, most of us don't eat a lot of whole foods, so we don't eat much resistant starch—about 5 grams a day, compared to 15 to 20 grams in a diet with little or no processed foods."

Seeing this lack in the daily diet, a food company decided to sell a powdered, fiber-rich resistant starch that you could *add* to foods.

Its source was a hybrid corn (a *non*-GMO corn, Rhonda was quick to point out) that was uniquely high in *amylose*, the dense, compact and therefore very resistant part of starch. (Typical starch is 25% amylose; this corn was 75% amylose.)

After harvesting, they treated the corn with low heat and moisture, to make the amylose even *more* resistant.

And then they ground it up into the powder that is now called *Hi-maize*—a fine, white, gluten-free, low-calorie powder that you can add to smoothies and shakes…stir into oatmeal or yogurt…or substitute for a portion of regular flour you use to bake breads, muffins or cookies.

The standardized powder was also a perfect way for scientists to study the health effects of resistant starch. Three hundred scientific studies later, there's a lot to cheer about.

This starch <u>lowers </u>blood sugar!

Because resistant starch is slowly digested…and only partially digested in the small intestine…and fuels friendly bacteria in the colon…it provides a wealth of glucose-balancing, fat-burning benefits—making it a super-food for people with blood sugar problems (or people who want to prevent them).

In the overweight, insulin sensitivity improves—up to 76%. The hormone insulin triggers the movement of glucose out of the bloodstream and into cells. But many of the nearly 105 million Americans with blood sugar problems have *insulin resistance*—their cells no longer respond normally to the hormone and blood sugar stays high. Resistant starch to the rescue…

In a study in the *Journal of Nutrition*, insulin sensitivity in overweight men improved up to 76% after they ate more resistant starch for one month. [1]

"The effect we saw in this study is very impressive—I'm a big fan of resistant starch," I was told by Kevin Maki, PhD, the lead author of the study and president and chief science officer of Provident Clinical Research in Glen Ellyn, Illinois.

Better insulin sensitivity in people with diabetes. In a study of 40 people with diabetes, four weeks of including resistant starch in the diet improved insulin resistance. [2]

It also improved fasting blood glucose…improved post-meal blood glucose levels… lowered total cholesterol…lowered triglycerides…and helped the study participants shed pounds.

Resistant starch works in healthy people, too. But you don't have to be overweight or have diabetes for resistant starch to improve your body's ability to handle blood sugar. Ten healthy men who ate a daily dose of resistant starch saw their insulin sensitivity improve by 33% and their body's ability to clear glucose from the blood improve by 44%, reported British researchers. [3]

Resistant starch for dinner, better blood sugar after breakfast. Another advantage of resistant starch: it keeps on working, long after your last meal. When people ate a dinner that included bread enriched with resistant starch, they had better blood sugar control after the next morning's breakfast. [4]

You'll feel fuller after a meal—and eat less the next day!

Twenty people who ate a high-fiber muffin made with resistant starch had far less hunger three hours later than people who ate high-fiber muffins with no resistant starch, reported researchers in the Department of Food and Science at the University of Minnesota. [5]

In another study, people who ate a meal with resistant starch ate 10% fewer calories over the next 24 hours compared to people who didn't eat resistant starch. [6]

Burn 23% more fat. Feeling less hungry…means eating less …which helps with weight loss…which is key to overcoming diabetes. And although there are no long-term weight loss studies in people regularly eating resistant starch, one study showed that people who ate a meal rich in resistant starch burned 23% more fat after the meal. [7]

The bottom line: "Scientifically, I compare starch to fat," Rhonda said, summarizing the research. "We used to think all fats were bad. Now we have sufficient scientific evidence to know that omega-3 fats are *good* fats. Similarly, we now know resistant starch is a *good* starch."

Also, Hi-maize resistant starch produces glucose-balancing results much faster than adding whole grains to your diet, she pointed out. "Research shows you would have to eat high-fiber bran cereals every day for six months to start to get some of the glucose-positive benefits that Hi-maize produces in six hours. And Americans are desperately in need of those benefits."

The resistant starch secret: It's a prebiotic

Some scientists theorize that resistant starch lowers insulin and blood sugar levels because it's a *prebiotic*—it provides fuel for *probiotics*, friendly bacteria in the colon. When those friendly bacteria flourish, there's less insulin resistance, chronic inflammation, and post-meal blood sugar spikes—three drivers of prediabetes and diabetes. (You can read more about the profound effect of probiotics on blood sugar balance in Chapter 4, "Probiotics.")

The friendly bacteria may also stimulate the secretion of several gut hormones—PYY, GLP-1 and GLP-2—that help control appetite and regulate glucose levels.

It also improves the way your body metabolizes fats and the pace at which your pancreas produces insulin.

This super-food also digests super-slowly, which naturally lowers sugar levels in the blood and staves off hunger.

"My blood sugar went down without medication"

Fran Stevens (not her real name) has firsthand experience of the benefits of resistant starch.

"I'm 76 and have had a lot of health problems, like type 2 diabetes, high cholesterol, high blood pressure, arthritis and being overweight," she told me. "Then Rhonda—a family friend—introduced me to resistant starch. I began adding it to my morning breakfast shake and to recipes for baked goods. Well, I was only a little plump—I'm 5'8" and weighed 179 pounds—but did I lose that weight fast! I was at 145 pounds just six months after starting the starch. And I went from a size 14 to a size 10, which is wonderful for a woman.

"During that same time, my blood sugar levels went down by themselves, without medication—and now they're totally normal! My doctor just shook his head in disbelief."

I asked her to describe her morning shake. "I take three tablespoons of resistant starch and mix it with protein powder, milk and some sort of fruit, like bananas or peaches," she said.

"I love to bake, and now I bake with resistant starch—breads, cakes, cookies, whatever. I haven't stopped eating those foods, but that hasn't hurt my blood sugar at all, as long as I make the baked goods with this product." (Her not-so-secret recipe: 25% resistant starch to 75% flour.) "My friends never know there's resistant starch in my cookies—they just think they're delicious cookies!

"In fact, I have several of my friends using it, and they're all telling me the same thing— their blood sugar and weight are both going down."

"And by the way," she added, "a lot of my other health problems went away. My cholesterol and blood pressure normalized, too. But my arthritis hasn't gone away. I guess there are one or two things resistant starch can't do!"

How to put more resistant starch in your diet

Rhonda recommends 15 grams a day of resistant starch for optimal benefits—three tablespoons of Hi-maize powder.

(You'll be pleased to know that even though resistant starch digests like a fiber, studies show that it produces no fiber-triggered bloating, abdominal cramps or gas, even when daily intake is as high as 45 grams.)

You can add the powder (which is widely available online) to smoothies or shakes…stir it into yogurt or oatmeal…add it to casseroles…or use it in pancake, waffle or muffin batters.

You can bake with it, like Fran does, using 25% resistant starch and 75% regular flour.

Or you can use 100% Hi-maize flour—the King Arthur brand—in any recipe that calls for flour.

You can also eat foods that have Hi-maize resistant starch as an ingredient. The website www.Hi-maize.com has a listing of the regional and national brands that incorporate Hi-maize resistant starch. Those brands include:

- Aunt Millie's Bakery (breads)

- Coborn's (breads)

- Wegman's (pastas)

- Ener-G Foods (a national brand with a wide variety of gluten-free, wheat-free and dairy-free foods)

- Nutrition First (bake mixes)

- Maninis Miracolo Pane (bread loaves)

- King Arthur flour

Anti-diabetes secrets in the next chapter…

- Remarkable scientific finding: spirulina might protect you from side effects of diabetes drugs.

- How to choose the purest, most effective spirulina—and the right dose for preventing or controlling diabetes

- More benefits from spirulina: healing liver disease…preventing vision loss…strengthening the immune system…and more.

EXPERTS AND CONTRIBUTORS:

Kevin Maki, PhD, is the president and chief science officer of Provident Clinical Research in Glen Ellyn, Illinois.

Rhoda Witwer is Senior Business Development Manager, Nutrition, at National Starch Food Innovation in Bridgewater, New Jersey.

RESOURCES:

To find a list of foods containing Hi-maize resistant starch, and where to buy Hi-maize resistant starch:
Website: www.Hi-maize.com

REFERENCES:

1. Maki, KC, et al. Resistant starch from high-amylose maize increase insulin sensitivity in overweight and obese men. *Journal of Nutrition*, April 2012, 142(4):717-23.

2. Zhang WQ, et al. Effects of resistant starch on insulin resistance of type 2 diabetes mellitus patients. *Chinese Journal of Preventive Medicine*, (2007) 41, 101-104.

3. Robertson MD, et al. Insulin-sensitizing effects of dietary resistant starch and effects on skeletal muscle and adipose tissue metabolism. *American Journal of Clinical Nutrition*, September 2005;82(3):559-67.

4. Nilsson AC, et al. Including indigestible carbohydrates in the evening meal of healthy subjects improves glucose tolerance, lowers inflammatory markers, and increases satiety after a subsequent standardized breakfast. *Journal of Nutrition*, April 2008;138(4):732-9.

5. Willis HJ, et al. Greater satiety response with resistant starch and corn bran in human subjects. *Nutrition Research*, February 2009;29(2):100-5.

6. Bodinham CL, et al. Acute ingestion of resistant starch reduces food intake in healthy adults. *British Journal of Nutrition*, March 2010, 103(6):917-922.

7. Higgins JA, et al. Resistant starch consumption promotes lipid oxidation. *Nutrition & Metabolism*, October 6, 2004;1(1):8.

Chapter 24

Spirulina

The color of healing is blue-green.

"Spirulina is a single-celled, blue-green algae that has existed on earth for eons," I was told by Suzy Cohen, RPH, a licensed pharmacist, and author of *Diabetes Without Drugs: The 5-Step Program To Control Blood Sugar Naturally And Prevent Diabetes Complications*. "If you viewed spirulina under a microscope, you would see the beautiful, bright, blue-green spirals for which it's named. The green comes from chlorophyll, and the blue from an exotic pigment called *phycocyanin*."

But its blue-green color isn't spirulina's best feature. That would be the *minerals*. "Spirulina is an *incredibly* rich source of the minerals that are a must for healthy blood sugar—for the health of your pancreas, the organ that produces glucose-controlling insulin; and for insulin sensitivity, the ability of cells to respond to insulin."

Two scientific studies back up that statement…

Lower levels of blood sugar and blood fats

In one study, researchers from India gave either two grams of spirulina a day or a placebo to 25 people with type 2 diabetes. After two months, those taking spirulina had across-the-board improvements in glucose and blood fats (lipids).

- Fasting blood glucose dropped by 20 points.

- A1C, a measurement of long-term blood sugar control, decreased by 1%, the level typically achieved by anti-diabetes drugs.

- Triglycerides fell 21 points.

- Bad LDL cholesterol, 7 points.

- Good HDL cholesterol rose by 1 point.

- Apolipoprotein A1 increased by 11 points. (Studies show this the level of this component of cholesterol is the most accurate risk factor for heart attacks and death from heart disease. As with good HDL cholesterol, an increase in apolipoprotein A1 is a sign of lower risk.)

"These findings," wrote the researchers in the *Journal of Medicine and Food*, "suggest the beneficial effect of spirulina supplementation in controlling blood glucose levels and in improving the lipid [fat] profile" of people with type 2 diabetes. [1]

In a similar study, 37 people with type 2 diabetes took either 8 grams of spirulina or a placebo. Spirulina lowered blood fats, and cooled inflammation and oxidation, the evil twins of chronic disease. Spirulina, concluded the researchers in the journal *Nutrition Research and Practice*, is a promising food for "the management of diabetes." [2]

Newest research: more protection from spirulina

New research in diabetic animals shows spirulina may also...

Protect your vulnerable kidneys. Japanese researchers found that supplementing the diet of diabetic mice with phycocyanin—the blue pigment in spirulina—improved five key biomarkers of kidney function. Spirulina, they conclude, may offer a new and effective way to prevent diabetic nephropathy (kidney disease), a leading cause of death in diabetes patients. [3]

Stop sugar-caused spikes in glucose—more effectively than metformin. When rats were fed high levels of sugar (fructose), their blood glucose and lipids spiked. But when they were fed fructose *and* spirulina, glucose and lipid levels stayed normal—in fact, spirulina worked *better* than metformin, the anti-diabetic drug, in controlling blood sugar. Spirulina, concluded the researchers, offered significant protection against fructose. [4]

Protect your liver from excess fat. Just about everyone with prediabetes or diabetes also has a liver problem—non-alcoholic fatty liver disease (NAFLD). This buildup of fat in the liver can cause inflammation and scarring, leading to liver failure or liver cancer. Brazilian researchers conducted a study to see if spirulina could protect diabetic rats from NAFLD. It did—and it did so more effectively than exercise. [5]

Boost the power of a diabetes drug—and protect against its side effects, too. The anti-diabetes drugs Actos and Avandia have been linked to osteoporosis. But when Indian researchers gave diabetic rats Avandia *and* spirulina, the rats' bones were protected. And animals receiving the drug and spirulina had lower blood sugar levels than animals receiving just the drug. [6]

Choosing a spirulina product; taking the right dose

There are a lot of spirulina products out there: powders and pills; spirulina-packed energy bars and snack bars; even spirulina chips, and tiny, crunchy, 1-calorie spirulina snacks.

How do you decide what to take and to eat?

Well, like any product, the quality of spirulina varies from brand to brand. But the best spirulina has several characteristics, I was told by Jennifer Adler, MS, CN, a certified nutritionist, natural foods chef, adjunct faculty member at Bastyr University, and owner of Passionate Nutrition, a nutritional counseling service in Seattle, Washington.

The taste is clean. "Top-quality spirulina *tastes* fresh," she said. "If it tastes fishy or 'swampy,' or has a lingering aftertaste, it's probably not a good product."

The color is bright. "Spirulina should have a vibrant, bright, blue-green appearance," Adler said. "If it's olive-green, it's probably inferior."

The source is pure. "The best spirulina is grown in clean water, in a non-industrialized setting, as far away as possible from an urban, polluted environment. If you can, find out the growing location of the product you're considering buying."

The price is, well, pricey. "You get what you pay for," Adler told me. "Good spirulina can be somewhat pricey."

One product that fulfills *all* those criteria is Spirulina-Pacifica, from Nutrex-Hawaii. It's been grown on the Kona coast of Hawaii—the sunniest coastal location in the United States, with a 12-month growing season. It's a unique strain of spirulina—*Spirulina Pacifica*—that is rich in disease-taming antioxidants. The spirulina is grown in water from a rainforest aquifer and the ocean depths, providing 94 trace minerals. The manufacturer uses a patented drying system to preserve the product's nutrients. And Spirulina-Pacifica is tested by an independent laboratory to confirm it's free of pesticides and herbicides.

"This is one of the most nutritious and purest spirulina products on the market," Cohen told me.

"A reliable, preventive, daily dose of spirulina is three to five grams, or 1 teaspoon," Adler told me. "A daily therapeutic dose—to control or reverse disease, including diabetes—is 10 grams, or 1 tablespoon."

As a health coach who wants to embody health himself, I follow Cohen and Adler's advice, taking three 500 milligram tablets of Spirulina-Pacific, twice daily. But pills aren't your only option.

Adding spirulina powder to your daily diet

There are many ways to include spirulina in your daily diet, Adler told me.

Take it straight. "If you want to get your daily dose of spirulina all at once, add a teaspoon or tablespoon of the powder to an eight-ounce glass of water or apple juice, shake it up, and drink it."

Put it in smoothies. "Add 1 teaspoon to 1 tablespoon of the powder to any smoothie or shake," she said.

Sprinkle it on food. "Believe it or not, my family and friends have grown to love spirulina popcorn!" said Adler. "It's a great conversation starter at a potluck." Her recipe:

To a bowl of popcorn, add one to two tablespoons of spirulina powder, three to four tablespoons of nutritional yeast, two or three tablespoons of olive oil, one-half teaspoon of salt, and one-eighth teaspoon of cayenne.

Add it to condiments. "Put one-quarter teaspoon in a jar of ketchup, barbecue sauce, mustard or salad dressing," she said.

Or you could snack on ENERGYbits…

Snacking on spirulina

"I think ENERGYbits are excellent for people with diabetes," I was told by Catharine Arnston, CHC, a certified health coach and founder and CEO of Bits of Health, which manufactures and sells the 1-calorie spirulina snacks I mentioned earlier in this chapter. (Catharine and I are both graduates of the Institute for Integrative Nutrition, which offers a 1-year course in health coaching.) "They are 100% spirulina, they balance blood sugar, and they are really filling.

"In fact, I think I would have become diabetic if I hadn't started eating ENERGYbits every day, because I had blood sugar issues, with my glucose spiking up and crashing down whenever I ate sugar. I have 50 ENERGYbits and 50 RECOVERYbits [another spirulina snack] every morning for breakfast with green tea. They keep me feeling full—and full of energy—until lunch.

"But I don't think you need to eat that many. I think the magic daily number is 30—that seems to give people blood sugar stability throughout the day."

Catharine points out that her spirulina snacks are extremely high in protein, which helps tame appetite and blood sugar spikes.

"Spirulina has 64% protein, and it's in a form that is far more bioavailable than the protein from meat—you get the sugar-balancing protein in your system within minutes, rather than within hours.

"That's why we sell a travel tin with our product," she told me. "You can fill up the tin, have it with you in your handbag or pocket or gym bag, and whenever you're hungry or tired, rather than eating an unhealthy snack loaded with sugar or carbs, you swallow 20 or 30 energybits, and you'll feel full and energetic, and your blood sugar will be balanced."

Catharine sent me a bag of ENERGYbits to try. I loved their nutty flavor, and they were every bit as filling and sustaining as she described. One downside: some of the algae stuck to my teeth. Not to worry, said Catharine. "While it's sticking to your teeth, it's cleaning plaque and removing bacteria."

That added benefit doesn't really surprise me, because studies show that spirulina can protect and enliven health in so many different ways...

More health benefits from spirulina

Healing hepatitis C. Sixty people with hepatitis C—a chronic and deadly liver infection—took either spirulina or a liver-cleansing herb. After six months, four of the patients taking spirulina had complete clearance of the virus, and two had partial clearance—a remarkable result. [7]

Preventing age-related macular degeneration and cataracts. Many studies show that the antioxidant *zeaxanthin* can help prevent age-related macular degeneration and cataracts, sight-robbing eye diseases that are common in seniors. When Chinese researchers gave a daily dose of spirulina to 14 people, their blood zeaxanthin levels nearly tripled—and stayed high for more than a month. "Spirulina can serve as a rich source of dietary zeaxanthin in humans," wrote the researchers in the *British Journal of Nutrition*. [8]

Managing blood sugar in HIV. Blood sugar problems are common in HIV-infected patients, because of the infection itself and as a side effect of anti-HIV drugs. In 16 HIV-infected patients, two months of spirulina supplementation doubled insulin sensitivity. [9]

Strengthening the immune system. 10 people who took spirulina for one week had a 40% increase in the activity of *natural killer cells*—immune system cells that battle cancer, viruses and bacteria, reported Danish researchers. [10]

More endurance for exercise. Nine men who took spirulina for one month had a 24% boost in their ability to exercise without fatigue. "Spirulina supplementation induced a significant increase in exercise performance," wrote the researchers in *Medicine & Science in Sports & Exercise*. [11]

Healthy seniors are even healthier. 78 people aged 60 to 87 took eight grams a day of spirulina or a placebo. After four months, those taking spirulina had stronger immune systems, less signs of cellular damage from oxidation, and lower blood fats. [12]

Fewer allergy symptoms. People with allergies who took spirulina had less "nasal discharge, sneezing, nasal congestion and itching," reported European researchers. [13] And in a study by researchers at the University of California at Davis, School of Medicine, 2 grams a day of spirulina calmed down the overactive immune system of people with allergies. [14]

Lowering blood pressure. In a study on 36 people aged 18 to 65, taking 4.5 grams of spirulina for six weeks lowered average blood pressure levels from 121/85 to 111/77 in men, and from 120/85 to 109/79 in women.

I think I'll munch on a handful of those ENERGYbits right now…

Anti-diabetes secrets in the next chapter

- The amazing, heart-healthy benefits of dark chocolate: lower blood pressure…lower LDL cholesterol…protection against heart disease…lower risk of stroke…lower risk of a second heart attack…and more.

- How to identify the types of chocolate that *really* protect your heart. (There are a lot of "imposters" out there, say experts.)

- The "just right" amount of heart-healthy dark chocolate to eat every day. (It's easy to overdo—and that's *not* good for you.)

EXPERTS AND CONTRIBUTORS:

Catharine Arnston, CHC, is a certified health counselor and founder and CEO of Bits of Health.
Website: www.bitsofhealth.com

Jennifer Adler, MS, CN, is a certified nutritionist, natural foods chef, adjunct faculty at Bastyr
University, and owner of Passionate Nutrition, a nutritional counseling service with six offices in
the Seattle, Washington area.
Website: www.passionatenutrition.com

Suzy Cohen, RPh, is a licensed pharmacist, author of the "Dear Pharmacist" syndicated column,
which reaches 20 million readers nationwide, and author of *Diabetes Without Drugs: The 5-Step
Program To Control Blood Sugar Naturally And Prevent Diabetes Complications* and several
other books.
Website: www.suzycohen.com
Facebook: www.facebook.com/SuzyCohenRPh
Twitter: www.Twitter.com/suzycohen

RESOURCES:

To order Spirulina-Pacifica, from Nutrex-Hawaii:
Website: www.nutrex-hawaii.com
Call: 800-453-1187

To order ENERGYbits, the 100% spirulina algae snack food:
Website: www.energybits.com
Phone: 617-886-5106

**To find out more about training as a health coach through the Institute for Integrative
Nutrition:**
Website: www.integrativenutrition.com

REFERENCES:

1. Parikh P, et al. Role of Spirulina in the Control of Glycemia and Lipidemia in Type 2 Diabetes
Melitus. *Journal of Medicine and Food*, 2001 Winter;4(4):193-199.

2. Lee EH, et al. A randomized study to establish the effects of spirulina in type 2 diabetes

mellitus patients. *Nutrition Research and Practice*, 2008 Winter;2(4):295-300.

3. Zheng J, et al. Phycocyanin and phycocyanobilin from Spirulina plantensis protect against diabetic nephropathy by inhibiting oxidative stress. *American Journal of Physiology: Regulatory, Integrative and Comparative Physiology*, 2013 Jan 15;304(2).

4. Jarouliya U, et al. Alleviation of metabolic abnormalities induced by excessive fructose administration in Wistar rats by Spirulina maxima. *Indian Journal of Medical Research*, 2012 Mar;135:422-8.

5. Moura LP, et al. Exercise and spirulina control non-alcoholic hepatic steatosis and lipid profile in diabetic Wistar rats. *Lipids in Health and Disease*, 2011 May 15;10:77.

6. Gupta S, et al. Spirulina protects against rosiglitazone induced osteoporosis in insulin resistance rats. *Diabetes Research and Clinical Practice*, 2010 Jan;87(1):38-43.

7. Yakoot M, et al. Spirulina platensis versus silymarin in the treatment of chronic hepatitis C virus infection. *BMC Gastroenterology*, 2012 Apr 12;12:32.

8. Yu B, et al. Spirulina is an effective dietary source of zeaxanthin to humans. *British Journal of Nutrition*, 2012 Aug;108(4):611-9.

9. Marcel AK, et al. The effect of Spirulina platensis versus soybean on insulin resistance in HIV-infected patients: a randomized pilot study. *Nutrients*, 2011 Jul;3(7):712-24.

10. Nielsen CH, et al. Enhancement of natural killer cell activity in healthy subjects by Immunlina, a Spirulina extract enriched for Braun-type lipoproteins. *Planta Medica*, 2010 Nov;76(16):1802-8.

11. Kalafti M, et al. Ergogenic and antioxidant effects of spirulina supplementation in humans. *Medicine & Science in Sports & Exercise*, 2010 Jan;42(1):142-51.

12. Park HJ, et al. A randomized double-blind, placebo-controlled study to establish the effects of spirulina in elderly Koreans. *Annals of Nutrition and Metabolism*, 2008;52(4):322-8.

13. Cingi C, et al. The effects of spirulina on allergic rhinitis. *European Archives of Otorhinolaryngology*, 2008 Oct;265(10):1219-23.

14. Mao TK, et al. Effects of a Spirulina-based dietary supplement on cytokine production from allergic rhinitis patients. *Journal of Medicinal Food*, 2005 Spring;8(1):27-30.

Chapter 25

Dark Chocolate

The super-delicious way to protect your heart

Believe it or not, I'm writing this chapter on February 14, the day millions of boxes of chocolates will be gleefully opened and happily sampled. All of those chocolates are likely to win hearts. But if the box contains nothing but *dark chocolates*—Godiva's Dark Chocolate Gift Box, or See's Traditional Red Heart with Dark Chocolates—they will also help win the war against heart disease.

<u>Scientists have found that dark chocolate—rich in health-giving plant compounds called *flavanols*—is a super-food for the heart.</u>

And that's a crucial benefit for readers of this Special Report. People with diabetes have a fourfold greater risk of having a heart attack or stroke. That higher risk translates into 85% of people with diabetes dying from cardiovascular disease!

If heart disease is your problem, dark chocolate may be your solution. Over the last decade, I've reported dozens of studies on chocolate and heart health, which show that eating dark chocolate (cocoa flavanols) can…

• Lower blood pressure

• Lower artery-clogging LDL cholesterol

• Increase artery-cleaning HDL cholesterol

• Lower the risk of forming artery-plugging blood clots.

• Reduce chronic inflammation, which drives heart disease

• Lower the risk of heart disease, and hospitalization and deaths from heart disease

• Lower the risk of stroke, and deaths from stroke

• Lower the risk of chronic heart failure

• Help repair the damaged arteries of people with heart disease

• Lower the risk of a second heart attack

How does dark chocolate love thee? Let me count the ways…

A flavanol is a plant compound that gives certain plants their rich colors—think the green in green tea, the red in red wine, the blue in blueberries, and the dark brown of dark chocolate. (White chocolate, in contrast, has *no* flavanols.) The flavanol in dark chocolate is officially called *flavan-3-ols*—and when it hooks up with your circulatory system, there's sweet healing in the dark. Flavanol-rich dark chocolate…

Triggers the production of *nitric oxide*, a molecule that relaxes the lining of the arteries (the endothelium), improving blood flow, lowering blood pressure, and decreasing the risk of heart attack and stroke.

Thins blood, helping prevent artery-clogging blood clots.

Delivers powerful antioxidants that cool chronic inflammation.

Helps stop "hardening of the arteries"—the calcification of plaque that slowly but surely leads to a heart attack.

Revs up your mitochondria, the tiny energy-creating structures in every cell (including the cells of the heart), helping your heart stay strong.

When it comes to your heart, dark chocolate is hot.

The proof is in the (chocolate) pudding

The key question is: Do all those heart-healthy benefits of dark chocolate apply to the arteries of a person with diabetes? Scientists have answered that question with a resounding YES.

Studies also show that chocolate may play a role in *preventing* diabetes in healthy people, and *stopping* prediabetes from progressing to diabetes.

Let's take a look at some of those studies and their results…

Boosts 30% better circulation within 30 days. In a study of 41 diabetes patients, those who drank a high-flavanol cocoa beverage three times a day for a month had a 30% improvement in circulation. "Diets rich in flavanols reverse vascular dysfunction [poor circulation] in diabetes," concluded the researchers in the *Journal of the American College of Cardiology*. [1]

Helps arteries stand up to sugar. Researchers in the UK gave 10 people with diabetes a big dose of glucose to send their blood sugar level skyrocketing. Before ingesting the sugar, however, half the study participants ate dark chocolate, while half ate chocolate low in flavanols. The chocolate-eaters had 26% better endothelial function and 44% lower blood levels of an artery-damaging oxidant. In other words, <u>a small "dose" of dark chocolate protected their arteries against the damaging effects of a big dose of sugar</u>! [2]

And chocolate works to protect you from excess sugar whether or not you have diabetes. In a similar study, "pretreatment" with dark chocolate protected the arteries of 12 young, healthy guys after they ingested a big dose of glucose. [3]

Reverses insulin resistance. Scientists in Italy studied 19 people with insulin resistance or prediabetes. The study participants ate flavanol-rich dark chocolate for 15 days and no-flavanol white chocolate for 15 days.

While eating dark chocolate, they had…a decrease in insulin resistance…better functioning of the insulin-generating beta-cells of the pancreas…lower blood pressure…lower total cholesterol…lower LDL cholesterol…and better circulation. [4]

In another study, Australian scientists analyzed the impact of "dark chocolate therapy" on more than 2,000 people with metabolic syndrome/prediabetes. "Daily dark chocolate consumption could be an effective cardiovascular preventive strategy in this population," they concluded. [5]

Boosts HDL cholesterol. Twelve people with type 2 diabetes ate dark chocolate for two months and then low-flavanol chocolate for two months. While eating dark chocolate, their HDL levels were 8% higher—a significant boost. [6]

Improves memory—because of improved insulin sensitivity. When insulin resistance is remedied, you're said to have better *insulin sensitivity*. And that's just what happened in this study…

Ninety seniors with memory loss and mental decline (mild cognitive impairment) drank a daily beverage with either high, intermediate or low levels of cocoa flavanols. Those drinking the high-flavanol and intermediate-flavanol beverages had big improvements in memory and mental functioning. They also had a big improvement in insulin sensitivity. And, say the researchers, the improvement in insulin sensitivity accounted for 40% of the cognitive improvement! (High levels of circulating insulin are tough on brain cells.) [9]

Prevents diabetes. A Japanese study linked the regular consumption of chocolate to a 35% lower risk of developing diabetes in men and 27% lower risk in women. [8]

Dr. Chocolate is in! But you have to make sure to eat the right kind chocolate and the right amount…

Your daily Dark Chocolate Rx

"Dark chocolate is the new, guilt-free super-food—the fact that it's so good for you is the best nutrition news to come along in decades," I was told by an enthusiastic Janet Bond Brill, PhD, RD, a nutritionist and wellness coach in Florida and author of three books on heart disease: *Cholesterol Down*; *Prevent A Second Heart Attack*; and *Blood Pressure Down*. (I first interviewed Dr. Brill about dark chocolate for my book *Bottom Line's Breakthroughs in Natural Healing 2012*, and am honored to feature her again.) But even though dark chocolate is good for you, you shouldn't overdo it.

"I recommend you eat no more than an ounce [28 grams] of dark chocolate a day, choosing a product with 70% or more cocoa, the component of chocolate that contains the heart-protecting flavanols," she said.

"But keep in mind that chocolate is a treat and certainly not a low-calorie food," she continued. "Most of the mammoth premium chocolate bars sold in the supermarket are 100 grams, with a serving described as three or four squares. That's about 40 grams—and that's much more than you should eat!"

Dr. Brill had another warning. "Watch out for health imposters, such as white chocolate, hot chocolate mixes, chocolate syrups and milk chocolate—all of which are *low* in flavanols."

Dr. Brill didn't recommend a specific brand. "Sample several dark chocolate products until you find out that appeals to you," she said. But as a health coach, I point my clients to three brands that I favor for taste, purity and potency.

One of my favorite dark chocolates are the one-ounce bars from Scharffen Berger chocolates—look for 70% Cacao Bittersweet Chocolate or 82% Cacao Extra Dark. (*Cacao* is a fancy name for *cocoa*.)

I also like Dagoba chocolates—they're organic and have a wonderful variety of flavors in 70% or higher cocoa. For my own daily, one-ounce intake, I eat 1/3rd of their two-ounce "Eclipse" bar (which delivers a whopping 87% cacao but still tastes great) or the same amount of their 74% cacao Xocolatl Dark, which includes chili powder. (It is a delicious variant of the way chocolate was originally served in ancient Mayan and Aztec civilizations: unsweetened and spicy.)

To maximize heart protection, check out CocoaVia, from the Mars Corporation. This flavanol-rich brand also contains plant sterols, a cholesterol-blocking compound. CocoaVia offers a wide variety of products, including *goodnessknows*, snack squares with added heart-healthy ingredients like almonds, whole grains and fruit.

(For buying info for these chocolates, please see the Resources section at the end of the chapter.)

Chocolate doesn't only come in bars, of course.

"Perhaps the healthiest way to increase cocoa flavanols in your diet is with cocoa *powder*, which is low in calories and sugar," said Dr. Brill. "Natural cocoa powders have the highest level of flavanols, followed by unsweetened baking chocolates, dark chocolates, and semisweet baking chips."

"The best way to get your chocolate is with unsweetened cocoa powder," agreed Deborah Klein, RD, a registered dietician in California and author of *The 200 Super-foods That Will Save Your Life*. "For maximum antioxidants, mix one tablespoon of unsweetened organic cocoa powder with a teaspoon of agave nectar, in a mug of hot water, with a dash of cinnamon—a delicious daily comfort drink! Not only is this great for heart health, but cocoa powder also stabilizes blood sugar levels, helping prevent diabetes."

For the best powder, look for the words "natural cocoa powder unsweetened" on the label. And look out for the word "alkali," which means the product was processed using Dutch processing with alkali—which strips cocoa of flavanols. You want a powder that was created with the Broma process.

NEWS FLASH: Just as my publisher was going to press, I learned of a new study on chocolate and diabetes, from researchers at Tufts University, Harvard Medical School and the USDA. Studying nearly 3,000 people for 11 years, they found that those with a regular, higher intake of cocoa flavonols had a significantly lower risk of developing diabetes. Chalk another one up for chocolate!

Anti-diabetes secrets in the next chapter...

- Why restrictive, pleasure-denying diets for diabetes almost never work in the long-term to control blood sugar—and the "mindfulness" diet that does!

- The key question to ask yourself right before you eat.

- How to know when you're *really* hungry—and when you're eating to soothe stress or relieve boredom.

- The no-willpower way to stop overeating.

EXPERT AND CONTRIBUTORS:

Janet Bond Brill, PhD, RD, is a nutritionist and wellness coach in Florida and author of *Cholesterol Down: 10 Simple Steps to Lower Your Cholesterol in 4 Weeks—Without Prescription Drugs*; *Prevent A Second Heart Attack—8 Foods, 8 Weeks to Reverse Heart Disease*; and *Blood Pressure Down—The 10-Step Program to Lower Your Blood Pressure in 4 Weeks, Without Prescription Drugs*.
Website: www.drjanet.com

Deborah Klein, RD, is a registered dietician in California and author of *The 200 Super-foods That Will Save Your Life*.
Website: www.livitician.com

RESOURCES:

For Scharffen Berger Chocolate:
In retail stores, they are available at Whole Foods nationwide. You can find a regional guide to stores that stock Scharffen Berger chocolates at: www.scharffenberger.com.
You can purchase their chocolates online at: http://shop.scharffenberger.com
To order by phone, call: 866-608-6944

For Dagoba Organic Chocolate:
They are widely available in retail stores nationwide.
To shop online for the chocolates, go to the website:
www.dagobachocolate.com

For CocoaVia Chocolate:
You can find a store locator for products or order products online at:
http://www.cocoavia.com

REFERENCES:

1. Balzer, J, et al. Sustained benefits in vascular function through flavanol-containing cocoa in medicated diabetic patients: a double-masked, randomized, controlled trial. *Journal of the American College of Cardiology*, 2008 June 3;51(22):2141-9.

2. Mellor, DD et al. High-polyphenol chocolate reduces endothelial dysfunction and oxidative stress during acute transient hyperglycaemia in Type 2 diabetes: a pilot randomized control study. *Diabetes Medicine*, 2012 October 6.

3. Grassi D, et al. Protective effects of flavanol-rich dark chocolate on endothelial function and wave reflection during acute hyperglycemia. *Hypertension*, September 2012;60(3):827-32.

4. Grassi D, et al. Blood pressure is reduced and insulin sensitivity increased in glucose-intolerant, hypertensive subjects after 15 days consuming high-polyphenol chocolate. *Journal of Nutrition*, September 2008;138(9):1671-9.

5. Zomer E, et al. The effectiveness and cost effectiveness of dark chocolate consumption as prevention therapy in people at high risk of cardiovascular disease. *BMJ*, 2012 May 30;344:e3657.

6. Mellor DD, et al. High-cocoa polyphenol-rich chocolate improves HDL cholesterol in Type 2 diabetes patients. *Diabetic Medicine*, 2010 November;27(11):1318-21.

7. Taub PR, et al. Alterations in skeletal muscle indicators of mitochondrial structure and biogenesis in patients with type 2 diabetes and heart failure: effects of epicatechin rich cocoa. *Clinical and Translational Science*, 2012 Feb;5(1):43-7.

8. Buitrago-Lopez A, et al. Chocolate consumption and cardiometabolic disorders: a systematic review and meta-analysis. *BMJ*, 2011 August 26;343:d4488.

9. Desideri G, et al. Benefits in cognitive function, blood pressure, and insulin resistance through cocoa flavanol consumption in elderly subjects with mild cognitive impairment: the Cocoa, Cognition, and Aging (CoCoA) study. *Hypertension*, 2012 September;60(3):794-801.

Chapter 26

The Only Diabetes Diet That Works

Relax and enjoy your meals
—because there are no "bad" foods!

There are a lot of diets out there that claim they're good for diabetes.

There's the vegan, or plant-based diet, featured in the bestselling book *The End of Diabetes*.

There's *The New Glucose Revolution for Diabetes*, which guides your eating choices using the glycemic index of carbohydrates (a system that measures how fast carbs turn into blood sugar).

There's the *The Glycemic Load* diet, which spins the glycemic index to take into account serving size.

There's *Diabetes: Fight It With the Blood Type Diet*, which instructs you to tailor your diet to the foods supposedly right for your blood type.

There's the all-raw diet, championed in *There Is A Cure for Diabetes*.

And then there's *The Sugar Blockers Diet…The Mayo Clinic Diabetes Diet…Atkins Diabetes Revolution…The Insulin Resistance Diet…Flat Belly Diet for Diabetes…The…*well, you get the picture.

As I just said, there are a lot of diets out there.

But there's a big problem with *all* of those diets—with *any* style of eating that says some foods are good for you, and some foods are bad for you, and you should never ever eat bad foods again.

Those diabetes diets almost never work—because almost nobody can stay on them for long.

Here's the typical scenario when a person goes on a "diabetes diet"—perhaps a scenario you know all too well…

You're diagnosed with diabetes. You're told to follow a glucose-controlling diet and are handed (or read about) a list of foods you should and shouldn't eat. Needless to say, you start out very motivated to stay on the diet because you're worried about your health. And you do manage to "be good" for a few weeks. But like most people, your willpower has limits. And pretty soon you're eating the same foods you ate before you had diabetes. In fact, you become so frustrated by all the dietary restrictions that now you're eating *more* "bad" foods. Is there a way out of this vicious, health destroying cycle?

Yes, says Michelle May, MD, founder **and CEO of the Am I Hungry? Mindful Eating Workshops, and** co-author of *Eat What You Love, Love What You Eat With Diabetes: A mindful eating program for thriving with prediabetes or diabetes.*

The key to managing diabetes by eating a healthful diet is *mindful eating*, she told me. It's about freedom rather than rules…insight and instinct rather than willpower…self-nourishment rather than self-punishment.

Here are some of the strategies for mindful eating that Dr. May has used with thousands of people who have struggled to manage their weight and control diabetes…

"Put aside any and all dietary rules"

Before you eat, ask yourself this key question. "People eat for reasons other than hunger," Dr. May explained. "Often the cues are emotional, such as loneliness, depression, anxiety, stress or boredom. These cues override our *internal* cures of hunger and fullness, and send you in the direction of comforting, convenient, calorie-dense, highly palatable foods loaded with fat and refined carbohydrates—the foods that are the least helpful for a person with diabetes. And because you're not hungry when you *start* to eat, you don't know when to stop. You eat until the food is gone."

Being told to go on a "diabetes diet"—or any diet—ignores those underlying cues, she said. "Put aside any and all dietary rules about what to eat and not to eat—they never worked and they never will!"

Instead, ask yourself this simple question before you eat: *Why am I eating?*

"Put a speed bump—a pause—between wanting to eat and starting to eat," Dr. May said. "Take a moment to realize what's *really* going on—whether you're physically hungry or responding to an emotional cue. If you discover you're not hungry, make a choice whether to use food to deal with something that isn't a physical need for food, or to redirect your attention to something else until you're actually hungry."

Learn to recognize the physical signs of hunger. How can you tell whether or not you're hungry? "Scan" your body—particularly your stomach—for physical signs.

"Get quiet for a moment," Dr. May said. "Scan your body from head to toe. Look for clues that your desire to eat *isn't* hunger—such as tension in your body, or pain, or worried thoughts. Also look for clues that your desire to eat *is* hunger—like a hollow or empty feeling in your stomach, or rumbling and growling. Do this body-mind-heart scan whenever you feel like eating, and also about every three hours throughout the day, to see if you're truly hungry and need to eat." (For complete instructions, read the Body-Mind-Heart Scan at the end of the chapter.)

Redirect your attention. If you're not hungry, one strategy is to distract yourself rather than eat, Dr. May told me. Go for a walk. Pet your dog. Take a shower. Brush your teeth. Do your nails.

Or, if you've identified the underlying emotional need that you're looking to food to satisfy—meet the need instead, in a small way. "Maybe you're overworked and stressed out and need a vacation," Dr. May said. "Take a few minutes to surf online and look at a travel site, or visualize being on vacation and resting in a hammock, or take a few deep breaths."

Learn to recognize when you feel full. Being able to decide not to eat when you're not hungry is one feature of mindful eating. Deciding to stop eating when you're comfortably full is another. "Mindful eating is not about *being good* but about *feeling good*," said Dr. May. "By identifying signs of fullness—and stopping when you feel comfortable—you'll have much better blood sugar control."

A smart idea for figuring out when you're full: Set an intention before you eat. Ask yourself, *How do I want to feel when I'm done?* "You probably want to feel good, energetic and satisfied—not bad, tired and stuffed," Dr. May said.

Don't be a yo-yo—be a pendulum. "Many of us are yo-yo dieters—we're wound up, tight like a yo-yo, either up or down, on or off the diet, restricting ourselves or overeating," Dr. May said. "It's healthier to be like a pendulum—with a gentle arc in the middle."

An example of how a "pendulum" acts: on a cruise ship, at the Midnight Chocolate Buffet, you enjoy a few bites of a few different things rather than gorging yourself.

"It's much easier to manage blood glucose when you have a smaller arc of behavior," said Dr. May. "But mindful eating is not about being in control or out of control," she emphasizes. "It's about being *in charge*, so you get to make choices about what you want to do."

And a recent scientific study shows that mindful eating *works* to lower blood sugar—just as well as the traditional approach of dietary restriction.

Mindful eating lowers long-term glucose levels
—just as well as dietary restriction

In the study, 27 people with type 2 diabetes participated in a mindful eating program, emphasizing eating in response to cues of hunger and fullness, and 25 participated in a traditional program of dietary self-management, emphasizing calorie restriction, the percentages of carbs and fats in an "ideal" diet, and portion control.

After six months, *both* groups reduced calories and their intake of refined carbs...*both* groups had significant drops in long-term blood sugar readings...and *both* groups lost weight. [1]

"The fact that both interventions were equally effective suggests that we should let people choose," said Carla Miller, PhD, an associate professor of human nutrition at Ohio State University and lead author of the study. "Mindful eating was very well accepted by people who had no experience with it," she added. "If mindful eating is appealing, then it very well could be the best choice for you."

"Managing my diabetes is so much easier."

Dr. May has guided many people with diabetes to eat mindfully and healthfully, rather than being a slave to restrictive dieting—and many have told her how much of a difference it has made in their lives. Here are a few testimonials...

"I was no longer going from one extreme to the other." "After I started checking my blood glucose, I became more interested in what causes it to change," said Paul. "One thing I noticed was that when I was too hungry, I overate, so, of course, my blood sugar spiked. I started paying attention to my hunger so I could eat before it got out of hand. This was a huge shift for me, because I was no longer going from one extreme to the other, which has made managing my diabetes so much easier."

"I stopped worrying." "When I was counting and measuring my food, I made sure to eat every last bite, but even then, I never felt satisfied," said Tess. "I worried about diabetes and food *all* the time. This preoccupation only made things worse. When I learned to eat mindfully, I stopped worrying and could focus on eating what I needed."

And here's a wonderful success story of a woman who uses Dr. May's methods for healthy eating—even on her birthday!

"I loved every bite." "Yesterday was my birthday and my husband brought me breakfast in bed—scrambled eggs and toast—so I didn't take the time to check my blood sugar," said Erica. "They had planned a potluck at work for me, too. It was going to be a good day!

"I was hungry again by midmorning. I tend to get a little anxious about that, but I reminded myself that hunger is normal. I needed a snack but didn't want to eat too much because of the potluck, so I ate one of the oranges that I keep at my desk."

"I checked my blood sugar before lunch and then looked over everything on the buffet table. I noticed that I was starting to feel uptight about all of the delicious things my coworkers had brought. I took a deep breath and did a quick body-mind-heart-scan. I was at 2 on the hunger and fullness scale, so I filled half my plate with veggies and salads and the rest with samples of other things that looked good to me. [See below for how to do this scan.] A couple of the dishes didn't live up to my expectations, so I just left them on my plate—and loved every bite of the ones that did!

"In the middle of the afternoon, they surprised me with a birthday cake, candles and all. I was only at 4, but it was yummy! About halfway through, I surprised myself by noticing I was satisfied—I just left the rest on my plate."

The Body-Mind-Heart Scan, a mindfulness strategy from Dr. May

"An important mindfulness skill is awareness of your physical sensations, thoughts and feelings," writes Dr. May in her book *Eat What You Love, Love What You Eat With Diabetes*. "Doing a body-mind-heart-scan will allow you to pause and observe what's going on inside right then. This skill is particularly useful when you feel like eating but aren't sure whether it's from physical hunger or head hunger. What you pause to become fully present and mindful, you can better identify your true needs."

The scan:

Pause: If possible, close your eyes for a moment. Take a few deep breaths and calm yourself. Be aware that being near food or thinking about eating might cause you to feel excited or anxious, making it more difficult to identify the signs of hunger. By taking a few calming breaths first, you'll reconnect your body and mind, making it easier to focus on important sensations and feelings.

Body: In your mind's eye, scan your body from head to toe. What physical sensations are you aware of? Are you thirsty or tired? Are you aware of any tension, discomfort, or pain? Does your body feel good? Ask yourself, *Am I hungry?*, and connect with your body by placing your hand on your upper abdomen, just below your rib cage. Picture your stomach. Think of a balloon and try to imagine how full it is. When empty, it's about the size of your fist, and it can stretch to several times that size when full. Are there pangs or gnawing sensations? Is there any growling or rumbling? Does your stomach feel empty, full, or even stuffed? Or perhaps you don't feel your stomach at all. Notice other physical sensations. Do you feel edgy, light-headed or weak? Are these signals coming from hunger, low blood glucose, or something else? This is a great opportunity to become mindful of your body's signals and reconnect with your inner self.

Mind: Without judgment, notice what you are thinking. Quite often, your thoughts will give you clues about whether or not you're hungry. If you find yourself rationalizing or justifying, *Its been three hours since lunch, so I should be hungry,* you may be looking for an excuse to eat. If you have any doubts about whether you're hungry, you probably aren't.

Heart: What emotions are you experiencing now? What feelings are you aware of? When you become aware of your emotions, you can better see whether they affect your desire to eat— and even what or how much you want to eat.

Final thoughts

I wrote *Defeat High Blood Sugar — Naturally!* with one goal in mind: to give you the information and ideas you need to balance your blood sugar and feel better.

If you don't have blood sugar problems, I hope you prevent them.

If you do have blood sugar problems, I hope you reverse them.

If you suffer from the complications of diabetes, I hope you quickly control and resolve your symptoms using the super-supplements and super-foods in this Special Report.

In short, I hope you master your health and feel great every day—and I'm sure you hope the same thing!

It's been a privilege and a pleasure spending time with you.

Be well, my friend!

EXPERTS AND CONTRIBUTORS:

Michelle May, MD, is the author of three books: *Eat What You Love, Love What You Eat With Diabetes: A mindful eating program for thriving with prediabetes or diabetes*; *Eat What You Love, Love What You Eat: How To Break Your Eat-Repent-Repeat Cycle*; and *Am I Hungry? What to Do When Diets Don't Work*. She is the founder **and CEO of the Am I Hungry? Mindful Eating Workshops, which help** guide participants to eat instinctively again, live a more active lifestyle, and balance eating for enjoyment with eating for health. To find out more about the workshops:
Website: www.amihungry.com
Phone: 480-704-7811
Email: mmay@amihungry.com

Carla Miller, PhD, is an associate professor of human nutrition at Ohio State University.

REFERENCES:

1. Miller CK, et al. Comparative effectiveness of a mindful eating intervention to a diabetes self-management intervention among adults with type 2 diabetes: a pilot study. *Journal of the Academy of Nutrition and Dietetics*, 2012 Nov;112(11):1835-42.

NOTES

NOTES

NOTES

NOTES

NOTES

NOTES

NOTES